Teaching
and Learning
in Nursing

Teaching
and Learning
in Nursing

A Behavioral Objectives Approach

Kathleen K. Guinée, R.N., Ph.D.

Macmillan Publishing Co., Inc.
New York
Collier Macmillan Publishers
London

Macmillan Publishing Co., Inc.
866 Third Avenue, New York, New York 10022

Collier Macmillan Canada, Ltd.

Library of Congress Cataloging in Publication Data

Guinée, Kathleen K
  Teaching and learning in nursing.

  Includes bibliographies and index.
  1. Nursing—Study and teaching. I. Title.
RT71.G86   610.73'0711   77-23402
ISBN 0-02-348360-1

Printing: 1 2 3 4 5 6 7 8

Year: 8 9 0 1 2 3 4

Preface

The roles of the student and the teacher have changed. Active participation by the student in the learning situation is now expected. The student and the teacher have become partners in establishing mutual objectives. The emphasis has shifted from the teaching process to student learning outcomes. As a result of this trend in education, objectives have become realistic. The learning situation is seen as having specific outcomes, discrete objectives that are attainable through specific learning experiences.

This book shows how nursing situations can be divided into component tasks, standards, and competencies. The student becomes familiar with the analysis of competencies by domains and levels of learning. Behavioral objectives are constructed. Steps in the selection and sequencing of learning activities are illustrated. A strategy of continuous evaluation is matched to the domains and levels of competencies to be attained. Individualized instruction is seen in the context of various learning activities. Special attention is given to methods of testing, aids, and resources.

Although the role of the student has become more prominent, it is stressed that the teacher's responsibility for consideration of the factors that influence learning remains unchanged. Hers is the responsibility for selection and sequencing of learning experiences and the environment in which they occur.

K. G.

Author's Special Note to Men in Nursing

It is recognized that men are playing an important role in the nursing profession. For simplicity of sentence structure in this book, nurses are generally referred to by the female personal pronouns.

Acknowledgments

Sincere thanks are due to my son, Vincent F. Guinée, M.D., for his assistance in the preparation of this manuscript.

Educators whose publications were most helpful include Benjamin Bloom et al.; Robert N. Gagné; Norman E. Gronlund; Fred S. Keller; David R. Krathwohl et al.; Robert F. Mager; Robert F. Mager and Kenneth M. Beach; Estelle Popham et al.; W. Popham and Eva Baker; Hilda Taba et al.; Ralph Tyler; James E. Weigand; the American Nurses Association; the National League for Nursing; and the New York State Nurses Association.

Contents

Chapter 1   The Role of the Teacher and Learner   1

Chapter 2   Derivation of Competencies.   13

Chapter 3   Analysis of Competencies by Domains and Levels of Learning   29

Chapter 4   Evaluation and Choosing Evaluation Devices   43

Chapter 5   Behavioral Objectives.   71

Chapter 6   Organization of Materials to Achieve Behavioral Objectives.   89

Chapter 7   Understanding the Learning Situation 111

Chapter 8   Making Contact with the Individual Learner. 131

Chapter 9   Extension of Learning Activities—Aids and Resources 167

Chapter 10   Grading—the Attainment of Behavioral Objectives. 185

Index 195

List of Figures

Figure 2.1. Sequencing Cognitive Information and Identifying Tasks. Step I: Analysis

Figure 2.2. Sequencing Cognitive Information and Identifying Tasks. Step II: Interpretation of Data

Figure 2.3. Sequencing Cognitive Information and Identifying Tasks. Step III: Application of Facts and Principles

Figure 2.4. Summary of Procedure Used in Sequencing Information and Identification of Tasks Contained in a Nursing Situation

Figure 2.5. Suggested Guide for the Breakdown of a Competency into Subcompetencies

Figure 2.6. Statement on a Patient's Bill of Rights, American Hospital Association, 1972

Figure 2.7. Some Activities in Everyday Life Converted to Competencies

Figure 2.8. Identification of Tasks in a Nursing Situation

Figure 2.9. Conversion of Nursing Tasks to Competencies

Figure 2.10. Common Activities in Nursing Converted to Competencies

Figure 3.1. Analysis of Competencies by Dominant and Secondary Domains

Figure 3.2. Levels of Cognitive Domain Analyzed for Observable Behaviors

Figure 3.3. Observable Behaviors in Nursing Analyzed for Levels of Cognitive Domain

Figure 3.4. Levels of the Psychomotor Domain Analyzed for Observable Behaviors

Figure 3.5. Observable Nursing Behaviors Analyzed for Levels of Psychomotor Domain

Figure 3.6. Levels of the Affective Domain Analyzed for Observable and Nonobservable Behaviors

Figure 3.7. Observable and Nonobservable Nursing Behaviors Analyzed for Levels of the Affective Domain

Figure 4.1.   Choosing Evaluation Devices for Measuring
               Achievement

Figure 5.1.   Competencies Analyzed for Cognitive
               Domain, Level, and Verb
Figure 5.2.   Verbs Representing Different Levels of the
               Cognitive Domain
Figure 5.3.   Competencies Analyzed for Affective Domain,
               Level, and Verb
Figure 5.4.   Verbs Representing Different Levels of the
               Affective Domain
Figure 5.5.   Competencies Analyzed for Psychomotor
               Domain, Level, and Verb
Figure 5.6.   Verbs Representing the Different Levels of the
               Psychomotor Domain
Figure 5.7.   Transformation of Competencies into
               Behavioral Objectives
Figure 5.8.   Sequencing of Subcompetencies
Figure 5.9.   Division of a Behavioral Objective into
               Subcompetencies

Figure 6.1.   Matching Guiding Questions, Tasks, and
               Intellectual Behaviors
Figure 6.2.   Two Methods of Sequencing Learning
               Activities—Guiding Questions and Intellectual
               Behaviors

Figure 8.1.   Planning Learning Activities to Achieve
               Behavioral Objectives
Figure 8.2.   Learning Activities and Domains of Learning
Figure 8.3.   Achievement of a Behavioral Objective and Its
               Competency

Figure 10.1.   Suggested Domain-Referenced Grading Form
               for One Behavioral Objective
Figure 10.2.   Domain-Referenced Grading Form for More
               Than One Behavioral Objective
Figure 10.3.   Sample Summary Record Domain-Referenced
               Grading

Chapter Behavioral Objectives

At the completion of Chapter 1, and given the information presented as criteria, the learner should be able to

1. Define correctly the process of teaching and learning.
2. Describe accurately how the philosophy of the institution is expressed in the education program in nursing.
3. Compare correctly the focus of goal-referenced instruction with the focus of the traditional approach in instruction.
4. Explain correctly the distinct advantages for both the teacher and the student in goal-referenced or criterion-referenced instruction.
5. Explain the influence of accountability in education on the behavioral objectives of the program in nursing education.
6. Analyze the teacher-learner relationship and state correctly the reason for recent changes in this relationship.

CHAPTER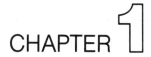

The Role of the Teacher and Learner

THE FRAMEWORK FOR TEACHING AND LEARNING

Definition of Terms

Teaching is a system of actions designed and intended to bring about learning. *Learning* is a change in behavior in individuals as a result of "experiencing." Teaching actions include the provision of learning experiences and guidance that facilitates learning, in formal situations, such as classrooms, and informal situations, as in health clinics, hospital rooms, and even patients' homes. The different aspects of teaching actions include planning materials and subject· content for presentation to learners, who may be students, patients, or others. The teacher is responsible for initiation action. The teacher sees and studies the teaching-learning situation, interprets and evaluates feedback and interactions, and makes an evaluation. This process involves constant observation and modification of behavior both on the part of the teacher and the learner.

Institutions Where Learning Occurs

Formally, we think of teaching and learning occurring in schools or institutions whose primary purpose is education. Teaching and learning may also take place in less formal situations in the community. In all cases, learning occurs within a framework of influential factors in the environment which affect its character, quality, and effectiveness in reaching the educational goals that have been established. This framework of reference encompasses the philosophy of the institution; the type of administration; the quality of administrators, learners, and faculty, types of patients, as well as individuals in the community, the physical plant, the equipment, and numerous other factors.

Policies and Philosophies of Educational Institutions

The philosophy and administration of the school, institution, or education program originates from the Board of Trustees and its members, who are expected to be acquainted with the interests and problems in the community. For example, a community may decide to organize a hospital for the care of the sick. Organization of a school of nursing may follow. The Board of Trustees are selected because they are thought to be representative members of the community and are expected to be acquainted with the needs of the people in the community. The bank manager who is a member should be acquainted with local economic conditions; the high-school principal should be acquainted with the social conditions of the youth in the community; the representatives from the health-care professions — nurses, doctors, and administrators — should be acquainted with conditions in their own fields of specialization. These people bring their beliefs and standards to the Committee and together they organize and write a statement of philosophy for the institution that represents the collective beliefs of the group. Such a statement of philosophy will be found in the college, university, or school catalogue. It serves as a framework within which the organization, school, or program can function with a purpose and objective. The school's policies and standards are outgrowths of the statement of philosophy of the institution. Administrators, deans, faculty, students, and patients contribute to it through their suggestions for changing and improving policy. This philosophy is expressed in different ways as varied as the quality of education, selection of teachers and students, protection of the individual rights of people, attitudes toward the value of human life, and the integrity of individual administrators and teachers.

Curriculum — The Implementation of the Philosophy

To bring about the possible implementation of the philosophy of the institution, teaching is the activity most commonly used. As a means to this end, objectives are derived that may include social, professional, ethical, and intellectual aspects of this theoretical framework. These objectives of the institution become the objectives of the curriculum of the education program. The curriculum is designed by teachers and students. It should reflect their personal, economic, and educational philosophies, as well as those of the institution. It includes all the planned learning outcomes for which the school is responsible, the attainment of the behavioral objectives, and the purpose of the program. It is clear why the success of the implementation of the philosophy of the institution is directly related to the quality of teachers in the institution.

The well-prepared and experienced teacher should understand that the focus of the curriculum will shift as the beliefs of the board members and other individuals and trends in society change. No specific template can endure indefinitely and remain effective. For example, as the public's concept of health changes from "freedom from disease" to a "state of wellness," so teachers must change curriculum, objectives, content, and learning activities to help students, patients, and others cope with health-related problems in their own setting.

RESPONSIBILITY AND ACCOUNTABILITY IN EDUCATION

The Teaching Process — In the Past

In the past, teachers and administrators of schools of nursing assumed responsibility for the education and development of students of nursing. However, in carrying out this responsibility, teachers and administrators were not asked to give an accounting to the community. The curriculum was designed to present information and selected learning experiences relevant to the objectives of the program and the school for the preparation of professional nurses. The focus of the program was on the teaching process, or on presenting learning materials to the students. The emphasis was not on learning outcomes. The statement of objectives was general and did not indicate what the student should be expected to be able to do at the end of the lesson or course. These objectives were not specific and did not indicate the behaviors that students were expected to achieve in a measurable form, or state how the learning outcomes or student achievement would be evaluated.

Few programs had plans for evaluation at the completion of a lesson or unit of instruction, according to predetermined criteria. In many instances, students did not know if they were progressing toward stated objectives until the final examination at the end of the semester. According to accepted practices in teaching, grades and answers to questions on the examination were often posted on the bulletin board outside the classroom, so that as the students left the classroom at the end of the course, they could confirm which of their responses on the examination was correct. There was little opportunity for feedback.

Focus on Learning Outcomes — The Behavioral Objective

With the emergence of accountability in education, administrators and teachers are now asked to give an accounting on the effectiveness of teaching and learning outcomes in the school to the administrative board and possibly to the community. The introduction of the accountability concept in education is relatively new. One well-known application was in federally funded programs that were designed to study student performance, or learning outcomes, as a measure of educational success. Other applications of the idea included performance contracting, where schools turned over the operation of a part of a school program to a private education company. The school would pay the company according to student learning as measured by achievement tests. These programs emphasized the use of systematic instruction, behavioral objectives, and criterion-referenced results.

The trend of accountability in education stressed the need for objectives that were more clearly and precisely stated and that could be used as instructional goals. In this way, learning outcomes could be defined more sharply and feedback could be improved. The demand for accountability of learning outcomes made it necessary for evaluation to be related to the objective or goals, and student achievement.

Behavioral objectives are unlike content objectives. They state (1) the actual behavior to be performed, (2) the conditions under which it will be performed, (3) the result of the performance, and (4) the criterion that will be used to evaluate the product or performance. Behavioral objectives provide the information that is essential for evaluation.

Responsibility Shared by Teacher and Learner

The term *accountability* raises a question regarding who is responsible and answerable for the learning progress of students. Those in charge of the education program are accountable to the Board of Administration, and the Board of Administration is accountable to its community. They must be able to document the degree of learning that takes place in the school.

Accountability places considerable responsibility on the teacher of nursing. However, the student is responsible for achieving the objectives. If the student is not successful in achieving her objective, then it is the teacher's responsibility to investigate such factors as the student's ability to learn, or personal problems that may be affecting her ability to learn. Criterion-referenced objectives provide measures and information that will help the teacher determine her effectiveness as a teacher, and help the student learn where she has succeeded or failed.

Accountability of the Teacher

Teachers are usually held responsible for the amount their students learn. But many factors impinge upon the effectiveness of teaching and learning. Learning as a product is not assured. Student learning outcomes in a school of nursing are influenced by many factors including the student's:

1. Acceptance of the subject content and the learning experiences provided by the school in the clinical nursing situation.
2. Ability to learn.
3. Own interests and needs.
4. Classmates' interests and attitudes toward nursing and care of people.
5. Past experiences and achievements.
6. Contacts with the entire staff of the college or school of nursing.
7. Physical environment, instructional resources, reference books, visual aids, and the like.
8. Home environment, including their family and other interactions.

It is generally agreed that the teacher should be held responsible for knowing the subject content in professional nursing, including knowledge of subject content from other subjects that contribute to the nursing content. Teachers should also have background information on their students that may be influencing their learning.

This can be found on the student's admission application and progress record. The teacher should have expertise in the application of principles of learning and an understanding of the factors that influence learning. She should have at her command suitable teaching strategies for the attainment of the objectives with appropriate variations to meet the individual needs of the students and the demands of the subject content.

Because the goal of accountability in a program is to improve learning and instruction, a teacher is responsible for participating in educational experiments in the school. Individual study and evaluation of her own performance as a teacher would appear essential and the teacher should be able to show evidence of the results. The utilization of this experimental approach requires a school atmosphere where teachers are free to explore and utilize different methods and materials for presenting subject content.

All teachers should participate in curriculum planning, including the formulation of the behavioral objectives of the program, selection of appropriate learning experiences, and an evaluation of the learning outcomes. The entire staff of the school needs to accept responsibility for the success of the educational program. The administration will need to encourage collective faculty responsibility as well as individual teacher responsibility. The professional staff shares responsibility for planning, implementing and evaluating the success and failure of the learning product, and making recommendations. The administrators and faculty who are given responsibility for the operation of the program will be expected to report tangible evidence of the degree of student progress toward the educational objectives of the school or program. Community leaders also believe that teachers and administrators should be able to present written reports showing the results of their successes and failures, indicating how they occurred and offering a course of action to improve their performance.

The aim of accountability in a program is primarily improvement in learning and instruction. Planning for accountability includes

1. Pretesting in all subjects.
2. Formulation of clearly-defined instructional objectives stated in terms of learning outcomes.
3. Selection of appropriate learning experiences for attaining the behavioral objectives.

4. Agreement on methods of evaluation for the learning experiences used in the attainment of the behavioral objectives
5. Construction and development of methods of evaluating the effectiveness of the learning experiences used to achieve the behavioral objectives at the end of units, levels of instruction, and at the completion of the program.
6. Construction and development of methods for the evaluation of the educational product or learning outcomes at the end of the program.
7. Recording of the achievements of students at the completion of the program including supportive data:
   a. Formulation of statements of acceptance of results, successes or failures.
   b. Formulation of statements of anticipated recommendations or suggested courses of action.
8. Provision of sufficient budget to cover expenses including evaluation processes.

Care must be taken in the application of the concept of accountability to nursing education programs. A faculty may limit evaluation to the acquistion of knowledge and omit the creative aspects of professional nursing. However, with the clarification of goals, objectives, and expected learning outcomes, students and teachers should have a good understanding of what is expected of them. In an education program, objectives and evaluation should serve to explain clearly and specifically what they are attempting to do.

THE TEACHER-LEARNER RELATIONSHIP — CHOOSING THE GOALS

The New Partnership

Teacher-learner relationships should be on a partnership basis. This relationship between two or more persons working together toward a common goal may be accomplished by involvement in the planning of the undertaking or learning experience. Most approaches to and methods of teaching allow for flexibility and the introduction of the partnership element; some approaches to teaching have a built-in factor that favors the partnership relationship. Regardless of the approach utilized, the learner should have a thorough explanation of

.the structure, content, and objectives of curriculum in which he is studying. The same approach applies to all learners. If the learner is a patient, his curriculum would be his total health plan. His objectives should be presented to him in nontechnical language suited to discussion. Unless the learner grasps the meaning of his objectives, he has not become a partner in the learning experience.

Goal-Referenced or Criterion-Referenced Instruction

Goal-referenced or criterion-referenced instruction provides an opportunity for teachers and students to develop a partnership relationship. Goal- or criterion-referenced instruction focuses on student learning outcomes. In this method, learner involvement is increased. Emphasis is placed on the objectives to be achieved by the student. The teacher assumes an indirect role. In using the partnership technique and behavioral objectives, the teacher and the student plan together the different phases of the teaching unit or lesson, such as previewing and evaluating films, or discussing and revising the objectives of the clinical learning experiences of the unit of instruction. By working together they close the gap between teacher and learner.

Goal-referenced instructional units are concerned with the observable behaviors the learner should possess at the completion of the unit. The goals are clearly specified. The teacher has a clear understanding of the competencies or behaviors the learners should be able to exhibit at the end of the unit of instruction. This will involve a designated time limit, possibly a semester, or three or four weeks. Goal-referenced instruction aids the teacher in selecting instructional activities. For example, when the teacher knows the desired terminal behaviors she can select learning activities that are more likely to help the learner attain her goals. Another distinct advantage of goal-referenced instruction is that the teacher can improve the quality of an instructional sequence during the term of instruction. She has definite standards, specified in the behavioral objectives, that she can use to evaluate progress toward the learning outcomes and she can modify the teaching strategy before the learner has completed the unit of instruction. Moreover, in goal-referenced instruction, there is a clear standard against which to judge the efficacy of the teacher's instructional procedures, and the importance of this cannot be overemphasized.

SUMMARY

Teaching is a system of actions designed to bring about changes in behavior or learning. Learning occurs within a framework of influential factors that affect the character, quality, and effectiveness of an educational program of an institution. These influential factors include the philosophy of the institution, the type of administration, the learners, faculty, types of patients, interests and problems of the community, and collective beliefs of those involved in the education program. The education program in nursing is sensitive to these influences, and the focus of the education program will shift as these conditions and beliefs change.

In the past, teachers and administrators of schools of nursing assumed responsibility for the education and development of students of nursing. The curriculum was designed to present information and selected learning experiences relevant to the objectives of the education program and the school for the preparation of nurses. The focus was on the teaching process. Objectives were stated but did not indicate what the student should be expected to do at the end of the course or unit of instruction. Certain influences in the community, including emphasis on the cost of education, helped to create the need for the introduction of accountability in education programs in nursing. This trend showed the need for objectives that were more clearly and precisely stated, and that could be used as instructional goals. The demand for accountability of learning outcomes made it necessary for evaluation to be related to the objectives or goals and student achievement, and behavioral objectives provide the information that is essential for evaluation.

A new teacher-learner relationship has developed since the focus has changed to criterion-referenced instruction. The criterion-referenced approach places emphasis on behavioral objectives to be achieved by the student. In the criterion-referenced approach, the teacher assumes a more indirect role and the focus is on learning outcomes not on the teaching process. This change in focus creates the need for teacher-learner partnership. The teacher and learner plan together the different phases of the unit of instruction. The teacher and student objectives are the same and both work together for the attainment of the objectives. The learner plays an active role and must produce evidence of personal involvement.

REFERENCES

1. Abdullah, F.,"A National Health Strategy for the Delivery of Long Term Health Care: Implications for Nursing," *R. N. Journal,* Vol. 5, No. 4 (1975), Convention Papers.

2. American Nurses' Association, *The Professional Nurse and Health Education,* Kansas City, Mo.: A.N.A., 1975.

3. American Nurses' Association, *Standards, Nursing Practice,* Kansas City, Mo., 1973.

4. Bell, Terree, "The Means and Ends of Accountability" *Proceedings of the Conference on Educational Accountability.* Princeton, N. J.: Educational Testing Service, 1971.

5. Dunaway, Jean, "How to Cut Discipline Problems in Half," *Today's Education,* Vol. 63, No. 3 (September–October 1974), pp. 75–77.

6. Dunn, H. L., *High Level Wellness,* Arlington, Va.: Beatty Publications, 1973.

7. Gagné, Robert M., *Conditions of Learning.* New York: Holt, Rinehart and Winston, 1965.

8. Gronlund, Norman E., *Determining Accountability for Classroom Instruction.* New York: Macmillan Publishing Co., Inc., 1974.

9. Guineé, Kathleen K., *The Professional Nurse: Orientation, Roles, and Responsibilities.* New York: Macmillan Publishing Co., Inc., 1970.

10. Keller, Fred S., "Good-Bye Teacher," *Journal of Applied Behavior Analysis,* Vol. 1, No.1 (Spring 1968), pp. 79–89.

11. Kemp, Jerrold E., *Instructional Design.* Belmont, Calif.: Fearon Publishers, 1971.

12. Lowenfeld, Viktor, and W. Lambert Brittain, *Creative and Mental Growth,* 6th ed. New York: Macmillan Publishing Co., Inc., 1975.

13. McCarthy, Joseph F.X. (Ed.), *The Training of America's Teachers,* New York: Alumni Association of the School of Education, Fordham University, 1975.

14. Metcalf, Lawrence E., *Values Education* (41st yearbook), Washington, D.C.: National Council for the Social Studies, 1971.

15. Schweer, Jean S., *Creative Teaching in Clinical Nursing.* St. Louis, Mo.: The C. V. Mosby Company, 1968.

16. Sward, Kathleen M., "The Code for Nurses: A Guide for Ethical Practice," *The Journal of the New York State Nurses Association,* Vol. 6, No. 4 (December 1975), Convention Papers.

Chapter Behavioral Objectives

At the completion of Chapter 2, given a situation where a male thirty years old was admitted to an emergency room in Hospital X and his condition was diagnosed as a fractured femur, the learner should be able to

1. Analyze the situation for its component nursing tasks, and justify the order and choice of questions used.
2. Decide on standards for these tasks in nursing.
3. Write a competency for each task. Criteria for 1, 2, and 3 established by the Emergency Room supervisor.
4. Select three tasks from a daily professional routine and convert them to competencies. Criteria based on information given in Chapter 2.

CHAPTER 2

Derivation of Competencies

IDENTIFICATION OF COMPONENT TASKS WITHIN NURSING SITUATIONS

Actual nursing situations are the source of information about tasks performed by nurses and learned by students of nursing. Tasks are derived by analysis of actual experiences in nursing situations, "on location" in the hospital, the community wherever nursing is performed. An analysis of abstract concepts, such as happiness, stress, pain, health, and other concepts relevant to nursing content will identify many pertinent tasks. This content is not static. For instance, some tasks previously performed by professional nurses are now divided among subprofessionals. As changes occur in nursing, the tasks of the nurse will change, and this will in turn affect the learning needs of students of nursing.

Tasks may be identified by application of a modification of Taba's method of sequencing questions according to their complexity of content. This method consists of three steps or levels:
Step I. Concept Formation. This involves organizing unorganized information by analysis

1. Enumerating and listing.
2. Identifying common properties, abstracting.
3. Labeling and categorizing, determining the hierarchical order of items.

Step II. Interpretation of Data. This involves forming generalizations or using inductive reasoning by

1. Identifying points, examining similar aspects of selected topics.

2.   Explaining items of identified information, comparing and contrasting, identifying cause and effect relationships.
3.   Forming inferences, implications, or extrapolations.

Step III. Application of Principles and Facts. This involves the process of deductive reasoning by

1.   Predicting consequences, hypothesizing.
2.   Explaining and or supporting the predictions or hypotheses.
3.   Verifying the prediction or hypotheses.

This method involves the use of the appropriate choice of questions to guide the learner in identifying tasks, forming concepts, interpreting data, and applying principles. Taba's approach helps learners form concepts of nursing. It encourages them to compare data and make inferences based on these data. The learner is guided in predicting consequences based on results of research or on principles previously developed in forming inferences and then verifying the predictions with new factual information. Figures 2.1, 2.2, 2.3, and 2.4 show adaptations of Taba's model to nursing education.

The adaptation of the Taba method of identifying tasks:

1.   Guides the student to take only the steps for which he is at the moment best prepared
2.   Increases the possibility of his learning success by focusing on activities that are relevant
3.   Facilitates the acquisition of gradually higher levels of learning
4.   Creates an awareness of progress among the class.

In analyzing the concept of Mr. Edward's nursing situation, which follows, questions are carefully worded, appropriate, and arranged in sequence from the simple to the complex. They provide for different levels of thinking and responses on similar levels of achievement of learning. These responses are influenced by the way the questions are worded. This strategy will break down the nursing situation into activities, or tasks, that are manageable, ranging from

[1]James E. Weigand (ed.), *Developing Teacher Competencies* (Englewood Cliffs, N. J.: Prentice-Hall, Inc., 1971), p. 148.

FIGURE 2.1. Sequencing Cognitive Information and Identifying Tasks

Step I Analysis

Guiding Questions	*Mental Activity*	*Tasks*
Describe the components or elements of Mr. Edwards' situation, including the equipment used.	Differentiate or separate the parts.	Enumerate the parts as you saw them (your own concept).
Based on relationships, what parts or elements belong together? Psychology, etc. Group on identifiable basis.	Identify common properties (abstract characteristics of parts).	Group these parts.
How would you identify or label these groups?	Arrange in order of importance.	Label or categorize the groups.

Adapted from E. Stone and S. Morris, *Teaching Practice Problems and Perspectives* (New York: Harper & Row, 1972), pp. 189–192.

FIGURE 2.2. Sequencing Cognitive Information and Identifying Tasks

Step II Interpretation of Data

Guiding Questions	*Mental Activity*	*Tasks*
Identify what you saw in the motion picture that related specifically to the administration of oxygen to Mr. Edwards.	Differentiate the elements of the concept you have of Mr. Edwards' therapy.	Distinguish or identify the parts or elements of the situation that related to the administration of oxygen.
Why were certain precautions taken in the patient's unit?	Relate elements in the situation to each other.	Give examples and relationships of identified information.
What significance does this have in the care of a patient who is receiving oxygen therapy?	Extend this situation to include implications.	Form inferences in this patient's situation.

Adapted from E. Stone and S. Morris, *Teaching Practice Problems and Perspectives* (New York: Harper & Row, 1972), pp. 189–192.

FIGURE 2.3. Sequencing Cognitive Information and Identifying Tasks

Step III Application of Facts and Principles

Guiding Questions	Mental Activity	Tasks
What would happen if certain precautions were absent in this patient's unit (physical characteristics of oxygen)?	Analyze potential consequences (recall possible chemical reactions, cause and effect).	Predict consequences or potential hazards.
Why do you think your predictions would come true?	Explain predictions and hypotheses.	What are the causal links leading to your predictions or hypotheses, positive and negative?
		Consequences: How may the outcomes be applied in other nursing situations?

Adapted from E. Stone and S. Morris, *Teaching Practice Problems and Perspectives* (New York: Harper & Row, 1972), pp. 189–192.

FIGURE 2.4. Summary of Procedure Used in Sequencing Information and Identification of Tasks Contained in a Nursing Situation

Analysis Step I	Interpretation of Data Step II	Application of Facts and Principles Step III
1. Enumerating elements of concept.	1. Assembling information.	1. Formulating generalizations.
2. Differentiating elements.	2. Explaining events.	2. Making predictions and formulating hypotheses.
3. Grouping and determining characteristics; labeling and arranging categories.	3. Comparing events and making inferences.	3. Applying outcomes to other nursing situations.

the lower level to the higher levels of implications and predictions in nursing.

The following situation is presented to the students in a motion picture.

Jack Edwards, a 58 year old foreman at Universal Shipping Co., noted the onset of a crushing chest pain almost immediately after helping to move a large crate. The pain persisted over the next half hour and he became weak and nauseated. The manager called the ambulance that brought Jack to the emergency room.

He was conscious on arrival, but pale and diaphoretic. The nurse attended to him immediately. She introduced herself and asked him about his present symptoms. She took his blood pressure and pulse, then notified the physician.

The physician examined the patient, performed an electrocardiogram, started an intravenous infusion, and ordered oxygen. Mr. Edwards was admitted to the hospital.

COMPETENCIES

Having identified the tasks to be performed, we must now match them with standards or criteria that can be used for evaluating the performance of these tasks.

A competency is a task performed to meet an established standard. In nursing education it is a nursing activity or task performed to meet an established criterion or standard of performance. Competencies should be taught, not the tasks or nursing activities.

Many combined competencies may be involved in one nursing activity, such as "making a correct nursing diagnosis," and a single competency for one learning situation may be one of many for a more complex nursing situation. Each teacher should write competencies for his own area of teaching. Figures 2.1, 2.2, and 2.3 are suggested guides. These descriptions should then be used, evaluated, and revised periodically to meet the needs of students and the needs of nursing. These same competencies may be common to different major areas in nursing. For example to "correctly apply the principles of sterile technique in a situation in nursing," could apply in almost any area of nursing, such as surgical nursing or obstetric nursing. The following are other competencies that are also common to different areas of nursing: "to read orders on patients' charts for accuracy, interpretation, and implementation;" "to construct an accurate and appropriate therapeutic nursing plan that will communicate the therapeutic regimen;" or "to correctly recognize how the loss of blood affects a person's physical signs." Competencies common to different areas could be determined by a subcommittee of the curriculum committee, the results could be shared, and the teaching of these common competencies could also be shared. The results should improve the teaching-learning outcome, influence the motivation of students, and strengthen the partnership relationships of students and faculty. It is important to note that just as there is a core of competencies common to different areas of nursing so there is a core of competencies common to other professions, such as communication skills, and also to general attitudes toward people. The selected bibliography includes the names of many authors in education who have contributed generously to this area.

The Subcompetency Relationship

Figure 2.5 presents a suggested guide for the breakdown of a competency, "Maintain a free airway by skillfully clearing the mouth and trachea of foreign substances, keeping the tongue in proper position," into subcompetencies.

FIGURE 2.5. Suggested Guide for the Breakdown of a Competency into Subcompetencies

COMPETENCY: Maintain a free airway by skillfully clearing the mouth and trachea of foreign substances, keeping the tongue in proper position. A limited breakdown of this competency to subcompetencies would be:

1	*2*	*3*
Apply knowledge of anatomy and physiology of the respiratory system, including structure and function and importance of the position of the tongue.	Demonstrate skill — clearing the airway while remaining calm, poised, and reassuring. Apply self-evaluation criteria on how to improve performance.	Explain correctly to the patient's family why he is being treated and the nature of the treatment. Apply pertinent knowledge of psychology and human relations.

AGREEING UPON STANDARDS TO BE APPLIED TO EACH TASK

The Criterion — A Level of Expectation

Nyquist suggests that the use of the word "standard" in education may lead to rigidity and tend toward conformity and sameness. He favors the word "criterion," because it connotes going beyond the established requirement for the performance. A criterion is used to arrive at a correct judgment. If the established criterion is the "minimum" requirement for performance of nursing it will be influenced by the prevailing level of expectation in the profession. This level changes with the level of knowledge, the supply of the profession's product, and the demands for the services.

Criteria for the performance of nursing care vary from institution to institution and according to supply and demand for nursing services, but because of the nature of nursing care, there is very little allowance for performance that is not correct. Whatever the nursing task or activity is, it is of vital importance and substandard performance should not be tolerated. This does not mean that in the past, substandard performance never occurred, but it does mean that if a person is ill, he is entitled to nursing care of an acceptable standard. If the student's activity is to administer a medication, there is only one standard, and that is the correct dosage of the right medication. This type of standard also applies when a nurse is to prepare and keep an area covered with sterile dressings or sterile drapes on patients, as those used in the operating room. Again there is only one standard or criterion. The area is either sterile or unsterile. It may appear that nursing is not flexible and should allow for at least 15 per cent error. We are inclined to think that the percentage of error would always apply to the nonessential part of the content of a course but there is no assurance of that and a patient has the right to expect care of the very highest standard. The Patient's Bill of Rights (see Figure 2.6) expresses the public's concern about the quality of nursing and medical care.

FIGURE 2.6. Statement on a Patient's Bill of Rights, American Hospital Association, 1972

The American Hospital Association presents a Patient's Bill of Rights with the expectation that observance of these rights will contribute to more effective patient care and greater satisfaction for the patient, his physician, and the hospital organization. Further, the Association presents these rights in the expectation that they will be supported by the hospital on behalf of its patients, as an integral part of the healing process. It is recognized that a personal relationship between the physician and the patient is essential for the provision of proper medical care. The traditional physician—patient relationship takes on a new dimension when care is rendered within an organizational structure. Legal precedent has established that the institution itself also has a responsibility to the patient. It is in recognition of these factors that these rights are affirmed.

1. The patient has the right to considerate and respectful care.

2. The patient has the right to obtain from his physician complete current information concerning his diagnosis, treatment, and prognosis in terms the patient can be reasonably expected to understand. When it is not medically advisable to give such information to the patient, the information should be made available to an appropriate person in his behalf. He has the right to know by name, the physician responsible for coordinating his care.

3. The patient has the right to receive from his physician information necessary to give informed consent prior to the start of any procedure and/or treatment. Except in emergencies, such information for informed consent, should include but not necessarily be limited to the specific procedure and/or treatment, the medically significant risks involved, and the probable duration of incapacitation. Where medically significant alternatives for care or treatment exist, or when the patient requests information concerning medical alternatives, the patient has the right to such information. The patient also has the right to know the name of the person responsible for the procedures and/or treatment.

4. The patient has the right to refuse treatment to the extent permitted by law, and to be informed of the medical consequences of his action.

5. The patient has the right to every consideration of his privacy concerning his own medical care program. Case discussion, consultation, examination, and treatment are confidential and should be conducted discreetly. Those not directly involved in his care must have the permission of the patient to be present.

6. The patient has the right to expect that all communications and records pertaining to his care should be treated as confidential.

7. The patient has the right to expect that within its capacity a hospital must make reasonable response to the request of a patient for services. The

hospital must provide evaluation, service, and/or referral as indicated by the urgency of the case. When medically permissible a patient may be transferred to another facility only after he has received complete information and explanation concerning the needs for and alternatives to such a transfer. The institution to which the patient is to be transferred must first have accepted the patient for transfer.

8. The patient has the right to obtain information as to any relationship of his hospital to other health care and educational institutions insofar as his care is concerned. The patient has the right to obtain information as to the existence of any professional relationships among individuals, by name, who are treating him.

9. The patient has the right to be advised if the hospital proposes to engage in or perform human experimentation affecting his care or treatment. The patient has the right to refuse to participate in such research projects.

10. The patient has the right to expect reasonable continuity of care. He has the right to know in advance what appointment times and physicians are available and where. The patient has the right to expect that the hospital will provide a mechanism whereby he is informed by his physician or a delegate of the physician of the patient's continuing health care requirements following discharge.

11. The patient has the right to examine and receive an explanation of his bill regardless of source of payment.

12. The patient has the right to know what hospital rules and regulations apply to his conduct as a patient.

No catalogue of rights can guarantee for the patient the kind of treatment he has a right to expect. A hospital has many functions to perform, including the prevention and treatment of disease, the education of both health professionals and patients, and the conduct of clinical research. All these activities must be conducted with an overriding concern for the patient, and, above all, the recognition of his dignity as a human being. Success in achieving this recognition assures success in the defense of the rights of the patient.

Criteria for Human Relations

Criteria or standards for interpersonal communication, or human relations, are of a more abstract nature but are just as important. For example, criteria must be evolved for the quality of communication with the patient's family when he is ill, or if death occurs. In determining criteria for the quality of performance of these activities in nursing, appreciation for the feelings of the members of the family is needed by the teacher and must be conveyed to the student. Empathy (which is putting ourselves in another's frame of reference so that we appreciate their thinking, feelings, and behavior) is essential to handling a situation of this type with calm and dignity.

JOINING TASKS AND STANDARDS IN THE FORMATION OF COMPETENCIES

Competencies in Daily Activities

It is important that tasks or activities in nursing are performed to meet established standards or criteria. A task is something to be accomplished. When it is performed to meet an established standard or criterion it becomes a competency.

Figure 2.7 shows some activities in everyday life converted into competencies. Figures 2.8, 2.9, and 2.10 present an application of predesigned questions for the purpose of identifying tasks, standards, and competencies on different levels of achievement, from the description of a nursing situation where the patient is having an anaphylactic reaction. The tasks being identified are activities that a nurse would be expected to perform or be responsible for their performance. (A professional nurse may assign certain activites to students or paraprofessionals in nursing and if negligence were involved, the professional nurse would be responsible.) On inspection

FIGURE 2.7. Some Activities in Everyday Life Converted to Competencies

Task or Activity	Standard	Competency
Drive car	safely	Drive a care safely.
Shoot gun	accurately	Shoot a gun accurately.
Speak French	with fluency	Speak French fluently.
Measure blood pressure	validly	Obtain valid blood pressure reading.
Sterilize equipment	without bacteria found on culture	Sterilize equipment so that bacteria will not be found on culture.
Recognize measles	differentiate from rubella	Recognize the difference between measles and rubella.

of Figure 2.8, it is evident that many of the tasks have subtasks, or in other words, prerequisite nursing tasks.

Figure 2.10 presents common activities in nursing converted to competencies. The information in Figures 2.8, 2.9 and 2.10 provides a guide for the analysis of descriptions of nursing situations, how to set up standards, and state competencies.

FIGURE 2.8. Identification of Tasks in a Nursing Situation

1. Define *anaphylactic reaction*.

2. Explain how this reaction may be prevented.

3. Demonstrate how to give a "sensitivity test."

4. Determine the time of onset of the reaction from the patient.

5. Describe the appearance of the patient.

6. Determine the inciting agent of the reaction by obtaining information about the patient.

7. Differentiate inciting agents according to expected anaphylactic reactions.

8. List the possible physiologic effects of anaphylactic reactions.

9. Determine, by examining the patient, whether a reaction is local or general.

10. Demonstrate how to maintain a free airway in a patient who is having an anaphylactic reaction.

11. Categorize drugs used in the treatment of an anaphylactic reaction according to specificity of action.

12. Make inferences related to possible reactions to treatment in this specific incident (care of the patient with an anaphylactic reaction).

13. Compare the underlying physiologic changes in anaphylactic reactions with the normal physiology.

14. Justify the choice of drugs used with this patient in this particular incident.

15. Predict the possibilities of similar reactions with other patients or people.

FIGURE 2.9. Conversion of Nursing Tasks to Competencies

1. Define anaphylactic reaction *accurately using appropriate terminology.*

2. Explain how an anaphylactic reaction may be avoided by *knowledge of correct information* on its causes.

3. Demonstrate how to give a subcutaneous injection *skillfully* and *accurately.*

4. Ask *appropriate* questions, listen attentively to obtain *information pertinent* to anaphylactic reactions.

5. Describe the appearance of a patient having an anaphylatic reaction by applying *accurate knowledge of observations* and make comparisons with the normal.

6. Determine the inciting agents by asking *pertinent questions,* considering possibilities, and making deductions.

7. Differentiate *correctly* inciting agents according to expected anaphylactic reactions.

8. List *correctly* the possible physiologic effects of an anaphylactic reaction.

9. While examining the patient, observe *accurately* the skin for local or general allergic reactions.

10. Maintain a free airway by *skillfully clearing the mouth and trachea of foreign substances* and *keeping the tongue in proper position.*

11. *Correctly* classify drugs used in the treatment of anaphylactic reaction according to specificity of action.

12. *Based on correct knowledge,* make inferences related to possible response to treatment in this specific incident (care of the patient having an anaphylactic reaction).

13. Compare *correctly* the underlying physiologic changes in an anaphylactic reaction with the normal.

14. Justify the choice of drugs used in this particular incident by *application of accurate knowledge* of drugs and expected reactions in this incident.

15. As a result of the *application of accurate research findings* on the incidence of anaphylactic reactions, predict the future occurrence of anaphylactic reactions in the hospital and in the home.

FIGURE 2.10. Common Activities in Nursing Converted to Competencies

Nursing Activity (task)	*Criteria* (standards)	*Competencies*
1. Address other professionals, patients, and members of their families.	Using correct forms of address for professionals, patients, and their families.	Use correct forms of address for professionals, patients, and their families.
2. Identify and interpret nonverbal messages.	Through sensitive observation.	Identify and interpret accurately nonverbal messages through sensitive observation.
3. Perceive the effect on a patient's emotions of an inability to communicate.	Appreciating the individual's need to communicate.	Perceive the effect of the inability to communicate on a patient's emotions, appreciating the individual's need to communicate.
4. Prepare a tray of instruments for a procedure.	Including all instruments usually used.	Prepare a tray of instruments for a procedure including all instruments usually used.
5. Administer medications to patients.	Within a reasonable period of time.	Administer medications to patients within a reasonable period of time.
6. Interpret the policies of the hospital to the patient's family.	Using understandable language.	Interpret hospital policies correctly and in understandable language.
7. Identify information related to a patient that should be kept confidential.	Applying hospital rules on patient confidentiality.	Identify information related to a patient that should be kept confidential by applying hospital rules on patient confidentiality.

SUMMARY

Tasks are basic components of competencies. Tasks in nursing are derived from nursing situations, concepts of nursing, descriptions of actual situations in nursing in hospitals, homes, and the community. These areas of study are analyzed for their component parts. This may be accomplished by using sequenced questions as a means of organizing unorganized material or information. The advantage of sequencing questions in complexity is that this strategy will not only break down the nursing situation or description of it into understandable order but it will also make it possible to set standards and form competencies on different levels of thought and complexity.

REFERENCES

1. American Nurses' Association, *The Professional Nurse and Health Education*. Kansas City, Mo.: A.N.A., 1975.
2. American Nurses' Association, *Standards, Nursing Practice*. Kansas City, Mo.: A.N.A., 1973.
3. Crawford, Lucy, *A Competency Approach to Curriculum*. Blacksburg, Va.: Virginia Polytechnic Institute, 1967, Vols. 1–4 (U.S.O.E. Grant No. OEG 6-85-044).
4. Davies, Ivor K., *Competency Based Learning: Technology, Management and Design*. New York: McGraw-Hill Book Company, 1973.
5. Dececco, John, *The Psychology of Learning and Instruction*. Englewood Cliffs, N.J.: Prentice-Hall, Inc., 1968.
6. *Glock, Marvin D., Guiding Learning*. New York: John Wiley & Sons, Inc., 1971.
7. Havighurst, Robert J., *Developmental Tasks and Education,* 3rd ed. New York: David McKay Co., Inc., 1972.
8. Kissenger, J.F., et al., "Teaching Medical-Surgical Nursing by Concepts," *Nursing Outlook,* Vol. 22, No. 10 (October 1974), pp. 654–658.
9. Klausmeier, Herbert S., and Richard Ripple, *Learning and Human Abilities: Educational Psychology,* 3rd ed. New York: Harper and Row, Publishers, Inc., 1971.
10. Lowenfeld, Viktor, and W. Lambert Brittain, *Creative and Mental Growth,* 6th ed. New York: Macmillan Publishing Co., Inc., 1975.
11. Milio, Nancy, "A Broad Perspective on Health: A Teaching Learning Tool," *Nursing Outlook,* Vol. 24, No. 3 (March 1976), pp. 110–163.

12. New York State Nurses Association "An Approach to Teaching Empathy," *The Journal of the New York State Nurses Association,* Vol. 6, No. 3 (November 1975), pp. 10–12.

13. Popham, Estelle, Adele Frisbee Schrag, and Wanda Blockus, *A Teaching-Learning System for Business Education.* New York: Gregg Division, McGraw-Hill Book Company, 1975.

14. Sanders, N., *Classroom Questions: What Kinds?* New York: Harper and Row, Publishers, Inc., 1966.

15. Sax, Gilbert, *Concept Formation in Encyclopedia of Educational Research,* 4th ed. New York: Macmillan Publishing Co., Inc., 1969, pp. 196–205.

16. Stone, E., and S. Morris, *Teaching Practice — Problems and Perspectives.* New York: Harper and Row, Publishers, Inc., 1972.

17. Taba, Hilda, et al., *A Teacher Handbook of Elementary Social Studies: An Inductive Approach,* 2nd ed. Reading, Mass.: Addison-Wesley Publishing Co., Inc. 1971.

18. Taba, Hilda, et al., *Teachers Handbook for Elementary School Studies.* Reading, Mass.: Addison-Wesley Publishing Company, Inc., 1967.

19. Thayer, V. T., *Formative Ideas in American Education.* New York: Dodd, Mead & Co., 1970.

20. Travers, Robert M.W., *Essentials of Learning.* New York: Macmillan Publishing Co., Inc., 1967.

21. Tyler, Ralph, "Behavioral Objectives," *Today's, Education,* Vol. 64, No. 2 (March 1975), pp. 41–46.

22. Weigand, James E. (ed.), *Developing Teacher Competencies.* Englewood Cliffs, N. J.: Prentice-Hall, Inc., 1971.

23. White, Marcha Strum, "Psychological Characteristics of the Nurse Practitioner," *Nursing Outlook,* Vol. 23, No. 3 (March 1975), pp. 160-161.

Chapter Behavioral Objectives

Given the following three competencies, at the completion of Chapter 3, the learner should be able to analyze each for dominant and secondary domains. Acceptable level of performance — according to information presented in this chapter.

1. Consistently exhibit interpersonal skill while questioning patients to determine their conditions and needs
2. Demonstrate how to give an intramuscular injection skillfully and accurately.
3. Assemble facts and differentiate between relevant and irrelevant facts.

Given the same three competencies, analyze them correctly for observable and nonobservable behaviors in nursing. Criteria as stated in this chapter.

Acceptable level of performance — identification of all the levels within each of the three domains of learning.

CHAPTER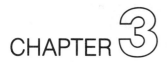

Analysis of Competencies by Domains and Levels of Learning

DOMAINS OR CATEGORIES OF LEARNING

When a competency for each nursing activity has been determined, the next step in the teaching-learning process is to decide on its domain or category of learning. This is necessary since competencies in different areas are developed in different ways. Categories or domains of learning are classified by Benjamin Bloom, et al., in *The Taxonomy of Educational Objectives,* as cognitive, affective, and psychomotor.

1. Cognitive behaviors involve the recall of information, and the process of analysis, synthesis, and evaluation.
2. Affective behaviors are described as emotive reactions or those that may be hidden from observation, but may be evident in values placed on what is being learned, or attitudes toward people and things. They are usually the direct results of cognitive or psychomotor behaviors acquired by the learner during learning experience.
3. Psychomotor behaviors are those requiring neuromuscular coordination.

Skills may be either cognitive or psychomotor. A psychomotor skill is the habit of making complex motor responses without conscious thought about the movements involved. A cognitive skill is the habit of making complex mental responses without conscious thought. An example of the first could be walking and an example of the second could be always beginning a sentence with the same word, such as "well." It should be noted that in nursing, psychomotor behaviors involve consciousness of thought.

Often all three types of behaviors — cognitive, affective, and psychomotor — must be combined to produce a competency such as "accurately writing a nursing-care plan." Writing the plan is an example of psychomotor behavior, recalling and evaluating the information is a cognitive behavior, and describing the condition of a seriously ill patient could involve affective behavior. A competency may also include behaviors in one, two, and possibly three domains. In any event, one domain will usually predominate. It is often necessary to emphasize one of the areas to measure achievement of desired behaviors objectively.

Analysis of Competencies by Dominant and Secondary Domains

Figure 3.1 shows an analysis of cognitive, affective, and psychomotor competencies by dominant and secondary domains. Two domains are identified and involved in each competency, one of which is believed to be more important than the other. In competency No. 5., "Demonstrate how to give a subcutaneous injection skillfully and accurately," the cognitive domain is dominant and the psychomotor is secondary. However, there is a less dominant element but also an important one, the affective behavior. For purposes of planning learning experiences as well as evaluation, it is necessary to identify and work with the dominant domain.

LEVELS OF LEARNING WITHIN DOMAINS

The Cognitive Behavior

There are six levels of learning within the cognitive hierarchy of behaviors:

Evaluation involves a decision or judgment of the value of knowledge, materials, and methods for given purposes. It may be quantitative or qualitative. Decisions are based on the extent that they satisfy criteria. The criteria or values applied may be those provided by the learner or those given to him.

Analysis involves the breaking down of knowledge, a concept, a topic, or a description of a nursing or other situation into component parts according to relationships.

Synthesis involves organizing parts, or elements, so that they form new complete patterns, ideas, or structures.

FIGURE 3.1. **Analysis of Competencies by Dominant and Secondary Domains**

Competency	Dominant Domain	Secondary Domain
1. Perceive correctly the effect on a patient's emotions of an inability to communicate.	Cognitive	Affective — Individual appreciation of mental distress associated with inability to communicate.
2. Accurately read patient's chart for information related to his nursing care.	Cognitive	Affective — Student appreciates need for careful reading for information and instructions. (Attitude toward work.)
3. Classify correctly drugs used in the treatment of anaphylactic reactions, according to specificity of action.	Cognitive	Affective — Application of knowledge and appreciation for the need for classifying drugs according to specificity of action. (Value placed on scientific knowledge.)
4. Effectively explain to his mother the medical condition of a child who is seriously ill.	Affective	Cognitive — Knowledge of medical condition.
5. Demonstrate how to give a subcutaneous injection skillfully and accurately.	Cognitive	Psychomotor — The injection is given automatically while consciously aware of reason for medication.
6. Dress in accordance with policy of the school of nursing and the hospital.	Affective	Cognitive — Application of policies of the school and hospital.

Application involves the use of abstractions in concrete situations such as nursing or other specific situations. They may be in the form of procedures, ideas, technical principles, and theories that must be remembered and applied.

Comprehension represents the lowest form of understanding. The student knows what is being communicated without relating it to other material or seeing it in its fullest meaning. It may involve restating knowledge in new terms, such as explaining and giving examples.

Knowledge involves recall of facts, principles, and terms in the forms in which they are learned.

Figure 3.2 presents levels of cognitive domain analyzed for observable behaviors as developed by Bloom, et al. Behaviors range

FIGURE 3.2. Levels of Cognitive Domain Analyzed for Observable Behaviors

Level of Cognitive Domain	Observable Behavior
HIGH	
Evaluation	Judge which data or actions are appropriate for a given situation.
Analysis/Synthesis	Gather facts from multiple sources and determine possible course of action.
Application	Use previously learned facts in a new situation.
Comprehension	Reveal understanding of material by explaining it in own words.
Knowledge	Recall facts and terms and discriminate among terms.
LOW	

From Benjamin S. Bloom, et al., *Taxonomy of Educational Objectives, Handbook I: Cognitive Domain* (New York: David McKay Co., Inc., 1956), pp. 62–187.

from the low level of knowledge or recall to the high level of evaluation or making judgments based on criteria. Previously learned facts are applied and utilized at the application level and above. This level of learning is significant to students in the professions. The application of knowledge to new situations is considered basic to the higher levels of learning, including evaluation.

Figure 3.3 presents observable behaviors in nursing analyzed for levels of the cognitive domain. Learning activities in nursing or behaviors are arranged in the same hierarchical order of complexity as the six areas within the cognitive domain. All levels of achievement are important and essential but teachers should plan for students of nursing to achieve their highest possible level.

FIGURE 3.3. Observable Behaviors in Nursing Analyzed for Levels of Cognitive Domain

Observable Behaviors	Levels of Cognitive Domain
	HIGH
Using data from observations of the patient and from his chart, make a nursing diagnosis.	Evaluation
Noting that three patients have developed a gram negative infection, report to the infection control nurse.	Analysis/Synthesis
Write the "night" report for patients on Unit X, in an acceptable form with correct data from the TPR and other records.	Application
Explain the cause-and-effect relationship between medicines that form a precipitate.	Comprehension
Recall the names of the categories of "cardiac" medications.	Knowledge
	LOW

From Benjamin S. Bloom, et al., *Taxonomy of Educational Objectives, Handbook I: Cognitive Domain* (New York: David McKay Co., Inc., 1956), pp. 62–187.

The Psychomotor Behaviors

In the psychomotor domain there are three major levels or steps *integration, application,* and *acquisition.*

1. Integration involves the formation of a pattern of action or behavior that becomes a routine part of a whole activity. The term *communication* is used instead of integration in many fields of education. However, in nursing, integration is a more appropriate word and describes what actually happens at that time in the process of learning a psychomotor skill.
2. Application involves different patterns of action done automatically while consciousness deals with elements of the situation, such as changes, or new elements.
3. Acquisition involves performance of the act automatically without involvement of consciousness.

Figure 3.4 presents levels of the psychomotor domain analyzed for observable behaviors. The three major areas are stages that the learner experiences or passes through. When the development of the psychomotor skill reaches the highest level, it is integrated into the nursing situation or becomes part of a whole activity.

Figure 3.5 shows observable behaviors in nursing analyzed for levels of the psychomotor domain. The descriptions of the behaviors in nursing should serve as guides to assist the learner in classifying psychomotor levels of observable behaviors. The psychomotor or motor skills area deals with the skills requiring neuromuscular coordination. Cognitive learning is present in the levels of acquisition, application, and integration. Below the application level, performance is without conscious attention. Skills can be developed and cultivated on different levels of performance, as has been noted. The degree of skill in the muscular action can be increased or lost, depending on practice and use. The performance of nursing skills requires conscious attention to the application of scientific facts and principles.

FIGURE 3.4. Levels of the Psychomotor Domain Analyzed for Observable Behaviors

Levels of Psycho- motor Domain	Observable Behaviors
HIGH	
Integration	Pattern of action or behavior becomes a routine part of a whole activity.
Application Adapting	Performs different patterns of action automatically while consciously deals with elements of the situation, that is, problems, changes, etc.
Manipulating	Performs different patterns of action automatically according to instructions without involvement of consciousness.
Anticipating	Performs automatically while experimenting with different patterns of action.
Acquisition Habituating	Performs the act automatically, with precision and speed without involvement of consciousness.
Coordinating	Practices the act until smooth patterns of motion are attained.
Modifying	Imitates the action while adjusting the position and movements to fit the pattern desired.
Reacting	Thinks about initiating an action and its elements, that is, start, finish, follow through.
LOW	

Adapted from Bruce W. Tuckman, "A Four-Domain Taxonomy for Classifying Educational Tasks and Objectives," *Educational Technology,* Vol. 12, No. 12 (December 1972), pp. 36–38.

FIGURE 3.5. Observable Nursing Behaviors Analyzed for Levels of Psychomotor Domain

Observable Nursing Behaviors	*Levels of Psycho-motor Domain*
	HIGH
The student nurse becomes able to administer injectable medication as part of nursing care of patient.	Integration
	Application
Give intramuscular injections automatically while consciousness is involved in preventing possible problems such as introduction of medication too fast or breaking the needle.	Adapting
Give an intramuscular injection in various sites automatically without involvement of consciousness.	Manipulating
Perform automatically while experimenting with modifications of technique.	Anticipating
	Acquisition
Give an intramuscular injection correctly without conscious attention and with precision and speed.	Habituating
Experiment with different movement until a smooth pattern is formed in the process of injecting a practice site.	Coordinating
Imitate the teacher as she holds the syringe, modify and adjust actions to fit the correct pattern.	Modifying or Adjusting
Examine and handle equipment and adjust it according to the instructions.	Reacting
	LOW

Adapted from Bruce W. Tuckman, "A Four-Domain Taxonomy for Classifying Educational Objectives," *Educational Technology,* Vol. 12, No. 12 (December 1972), pp. 36–38.

The Affective Behaviors

In the affective domain the high level of responding is subdivided into two levels, namely, *internalizing* and *organizing*. The low level of responding is subdivided into three levels, namely, *valuing, responding,* and *receiving.*

The following explanations are suggested as guides to assist the learner in classifying affective behaviors according to level. The affective hierarchy of behaviors is listed in descending order of complexity:

1. Internalizing is an observable behavior. The learner consistently acts in accordance with the values he accepts and his behavior becomes part of his personality.
2. Organizing is a nonobservable behavior. From this point, the learner enters the high level of responding by planning and organizing his values, determining interrelations, and accepting some as dominant.
3. Valuing is a nonobservable behavior. It involves analyzing the worth of the activity and formulating attitudes.
4. Responding is an observable behavior in which the learner reacts to an event through some form of participation.
5. Receiving is a nonobservable behavior and means that the learner or student is aware of the behavior and is willing to pay attention to it.

If we consider the levels of affective behaviors, from receiving to internalizing, on a continuum, there is an emotional quality that ranges from awareness to internalization, when the phenomenon becomes a part of one's personality. At the lowest level, emotion plays a small part; at the middle it is recognized as a critical part of the behavior. The title "valuing" indicates a point at which the control is becoming internalized. As the behavior becomes internalized and routine, the emotion decreases.

Figure 3.6 presents levels of the affective domain analyzed for observable and nonobservable behaviors as developed by Krathwohl, et al. Receiving is shown as the lowest level of behavioral change, when the learner begins to think about the behavior to be developed. Organizing occurs when the student begins to establish

FIGURE 3.6. **Levels of the Affective Domain Analyzed for Observable and Nonobservable Behaviors**

Levels of Affective Domain	Observable and Nonobservable Behaviors

HIGH

High Levels of Responding

    Internalizing — Observable — Reveals by consistent automatic responses to situations that affective behavior is a part of general behavior pattern.

    Organizing — Nonobservable — Recognizes value of behavior and establishes some system of exhibiting desired behavior.

Low Levels of Responding

    Valuing — Nonobservable — Sees the value of this attitude or trait and recognizes how it can be important.

    Responding — Observable — Reacts by answering questions, participating in discussions, working with others, and following instructions.

    Receiving — Nonobservable — Begins to think about behavior to be developed.

LOW

Adapted from David R. Krathwohl, et al., *Taxonomy of Educational Objectives, Handbook II: Affective Domain* (New York: David McKay Co., Inc., 1964), p. 95.

some system for exhibiting the desired behavior. At the internalizing level, consistent automatic responses are revealed as part of a general behavior pattern of the personality.

Figure 3.7 shows observable and nonobservable nursing behaviors analyzed for levels of the affective domain. The high level of responding is subdivided into two levels of responding, namely, internalizing and organizing. The low level of responding is subdivided into three levels of responding: valuing, responding, and receiving.

FIGURE 3.7. Observable and Nonobservable Nursing Behaviors Analyzed for Levels of the Affective Domain

Observable and Nonobservable Behaviors in Nursing	Levels of Affective Domain
	HIGH
Observable — Vauing the desirability of consideration of the patient, obtain more comfortable chairs for the clinic reception area.	Internalizing or characterization
Nonobservable — Recognizing the desirability of consideration for the patient, plan to make a clinic reception area more pleasant.	Organizing
Nonobservable — Become aware of the desirable attitude of consideration for patients — but no action is considered.	Valuing
Observable — Discuss with others the need for consideration of patients.	Responding
Nonobservable — An interest in the consideration of the rights of patients is noted.	Receiving
	LOW

Adapted from David R. Krathwohl, et al., *Taxonomy of Educational Objectives, Handbook II: Affective Domain* (New York: David McKay Co., Inc., 1964), p. 95.

SUMMARY

In the teaching-learning process, when a competency for a task has been determined, it is then necessary to categorize it into a domain of learning. Bloom, et al., classified categories of learning as cognitive, affective, and psychomotor. The utilization of all three categories is necessary, since competencies in different domains are developed in different ways. The cognitive behaviors involve recall of information, and the process of analysis, synthesis, and evaluation. Affective behaviors are described as those that may be hidden from observation. Psychomotor behaviors may include complex motor responses without conscious thought, such as walking. However, in nursing, psychomotor behaviors are those that involve consciousness of thought. A competency may include behaviors from one, two, or three domains. The contribution of one domain will usually predominate. It is necessary to emphasize the dominant domain to measure achievement of desired skills and objectives.

For purposes of evaluation, the determination of observable behaviors and levels of learning within domains are necessary. For example, in the cognitive domain, knowledge, comprehension, application, analysis, synthesis, and evaluation comprise the range of behaviors, in ascending order.

All levels of achievement are important and essential, but teachers should plan for students of nursing to achieve their highest possible level. In the psychomotor domain the three major stages of learning within the domain — integration, application, and acquisition — are generally utilized in teaching. In the affective domain the hierarchy of behaviors ranges from merely being aware of a behavior to actually incorporating the behavior into one's personality. Emotional involvement in this process increases until the learner accepts the behavior as her own.

REFERENCES

1. Banghart, Frank, *Educational Systems Analysis*. New York: Macmillan Publishing Co., Inc., 1969.

2. Davies, Ivor K., *Compentency Based Learning: Technology, Management and Design*. New York: McGraw-Hill Book Company, 1973.

3. Dececco, John, *The Psychology of Learning and Instruction*. Englewood Cliffs, N.J.: Prentice-Hall, Inc., 1968.

4. Dunaway, Jean, "How to Cut Discipline Problems in Half," *Today's Education*, Vol. 63, No. 3 (September–October 1974), pp. 75–77.

5. Gronlund, Norman E., *Stating Behavioral Objectives for Classroom Instruction*. New York: Macmillan Publishing Co., Inc., 1970.

6. Harbeck, Mary B., "Instructional Objectives in the Affective Domain," *Educational Technology*, Vol. 10, No. 1 (January 1970), pp. 49–52.

7. Klausmeier, Herbert S., and Richard Ripple, *Learning and Human Abilities: Educational Psychology*, 3rd ed. New York: Harper and Row, Publishers, Inc., 1971.

8. Krathwohl, David R., et al., *Taxonomy of Educational Objectives, Handbook II: Affective Domain*. New York: David McKay Co., Inc. 1964.

9. Levinson, Harry, "Appraisal of What Performance?" *Harvard Business Review*, Vol. 54, No. 4 (July–August 1976), pp. 30-36.

10. Mager, Robert F., *Developing Attitude Toward Learning.* Belmont, Calif.: Fearon Publishers, 1968.

11. Mager, Robert, and Peter Pipe, *Analyzing Performance Problems, or "You Really Oughta Wanna."* Belmont, Calif.: Fearon Publishers/Lear Siegler, Inc., 1970.

12. McAshan, H.H., *Writing Behavioral Objectives.* New York: Harper and Row, Publishers, Inc., 1970.

13. Plowman, Paul D., *Behavioral Objectives.* Chicago, Ill.: Science Research Associates, Inc., 1971.

14. Popham, Estelle, Adele Frisbee Schrag, and Wanda Blockus, *A Teaching-Learning System for Business Education.* New York: Gregg Division, McGraw-Hill Book Company, 1975.

15. Popham, James W., and Eva I. Baker, *Planning Instructional Sequence.* Englewood Cliffs, N.J.: Prentice-Hall, Inc., 1970.

16. Popham, James W., *Criterion-Referenced Measurement: An Introduction.* Englewood Cliffs, N.J.: Educational Technology Publications, Inc., 1971.

17. Simon, Sidney B., Leland Howe, and Howard Kirschenbaum, *Values Clarification: A Handbook of Practical Strategies for Teachers and Students.* New York: Hart Publishing Company, 1972.

18. Skinner, B.F., *The Technology of Teaching.* New York: Appleton-Century-Crofts, 1968.

19. Sward, Kathleen M., "The Code for Nurses: A Guide for Ethical Practice," *The Journal of the New York State Nurses Association,* Vol. 6, No. 4 (December 1975), Convention Papers.

20. Taba, Hilda, et al., *A Teacher Handbook of Elementary Social Studies: An Inductive Approach,* 2nd ed. Reading, Mass.: Addison-Wesley Publishing Co., Inc., 1971.

21. Thayer, V.T., *Formative Ideas in American Education.* New York: Dodd, Mead & Co., 1970.

22. Tuckman, Bruce W., "A Four-Domain Taxonomy for Classifying Educational Tasks and Objectives," *Educational Technology,* Vol. 12, No. 12 (December 1972), pp. 36–38.

23. Tyler, Ralph, "Behavioral Objectives," *Today's Education,* Vol. 64, No. 2. (March 1975), pp. 41–46.

24. Wright, Kenneth B., Rupert N. Evans, Edward F. Mackin, and Garth M. Mangum, *Career Education. What It Is and How To Do It.* Salt Lake City, Utah: Olympus Publishing Company, 1972.

Chapter Behavioral Objectives

Given the information in Chapter 4, and using it as criteria, the learner should be able to

1. Describe accurately the function of a competency in evaluating achievement toward behavioral objectives.
2. Compare the meaning of the terms *measurement* and *evaluation*.
3. Correctly differentiate between norm-referenced and criterion-referenced measures.
4. Given three competencies from Figure 4.1, correctly decide the dominant domain and the level of learning that should be achieved for each of the competencies in nursing, according to information given in this chapter.
5. Identify correctly the characteristics of the levels of learning within the affective and psychomotor domains.

CHAPTER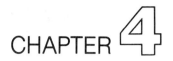

Evaluation and Choosing Evaluation Devices

EVALUATION IN NURSING EDUCATION

Evaluation is the concern of all those who participate in the educational program in nursing. Evaluation is a familiar term to both students and faculty. It implies a measurement. Measurement is the placement or position of a score achieved by the student on a predetermined rating scale, such as 1 to 100. Evaluation is the interpretation of the value of the position of the score on that particular scale. Students entering a school of nursing are acclimated to different types of tests in high school before entering college. Students entering nursing education programs usually complete the prenursing examinations and college entrance and aptitude tests required for admission to the school of nursing. They are familiar with the system of measurement and evaluation in these tests.

When students are admitted to a school of nursing, they will become familiar with the purpose and objectives of the school and the type of nurse the school plans to graduate. The objectives describe the characteristics of a person whom it is thought will function effectively as a nurse and as a representative professional person from the particular school. The attainment of these qualities is approached by means of clearly defined objectives, such as "A graduate of the program should consistently exhibit ethical standards of behavior." Since this objective is general, it will be broken down into its contributing subdivisions so that it can be approached by participation in many different learning activities.

Since the objectives are broad, evaluation in nursing education must be comprehensive, and designed to contribute to the objectives of the school and to the objectives of the curriculum. There will be a need for pretesting and retesting and for recorded evaluations by different faculty and other qualified people. The evaluations should be of activities that are natural and expected to be performed in nursing situations. Evaluations should be specific enough for a valid interpretation to be made. The value of comprehensive evaluation is lost unless detailed records are made and kept available in the student's cumulative record.

The Purpose of Evaluation

Evaluation is a basic element in a teaching-learning program in nursing education. It is used to determine how much the student has achieved and to find out if she possesses the foundation for new knowledge. This is necessary since advanced theories are built upon less complex theories. Evaluation measures keep the student informed on her progress toward the objectives. This information obtained (called *feedback*) from the evaluation is essential for making revisions in the educational program and revitalizing its content. For instance, an analysis of the results of tests or other evaluation measures, such as observations of individual performance made while the student participates in clinical nursing, can indicate deficiencies in the learning sequence and the need for corrections. The sequence of learning experiences in the clinical area may need to be changed to make the learning experiences more interesting or less difficult.

For the teacher, evaluation of the student's achievement and progress provides information that is valuable in guiding and directing current teaching. It offers opportunities to recognize and reinforce the successes of students and to utilize them as motivating forces. The identification of errors and inquiry into the reasons they occurred can help the teacher evaluate her own teaching. For instance, the error may have occurred because the instructional objectives were not clearly explained, or the learning activities were not related to the objectives, or were too limited in their resemblance to real-life situations in nursing.

Evaluation can be used by the teacher as a subject for communication to inform the student of her progress. Evaluation may also be used as a subject for communication with parents, to inform them of the rate and pattern of progress of their son or daughter in the program of nursing. Parents are interested in the achievement of their adult sons and daughters, not only for personal but also for economic reasons. The high cost of education has introduced a note of accountability in the parent-teacher relationship.

Evaluation provides information that is valuable for short- or long-term planning for continuing education. The accumulation of this information and the analysis of it largely determines the individual nurse's plans for continuing education after graduation. It may be a determining factor in the admission of a nurse to a graduate program of nursing or it may be a direct influence on the type of specialty the nurse will pursue. This background of information shows the rate and pattern of the student's progress and may be utilized throughout her professional life in such instances as changing positions or applying for scholarship aid.

Validity of Education Measures

Validity of content in measurement is obtained by using an adequately large number of test items for each learning outcome. A test is considered valid when it measures what it is supposed to measure. Each test item should be designed to measure the specific behavior described in the competency of the learning outcome. The number of test items should be adequate, but need not be exhaustive. When interpretations are made on small numbers of test items, decisions should be tentative, and supplementary evaluations, such as observation of individual performance, or norm-referenced tests, should be utilized as well.

The selection of the evaluation device is important. For instance, if the purpose of the test is to measure the student's knowledge of scientific information applicable to drainage of cavities of the body and it asks questions related to the effects of insulin on diabetes mellitus, the test will lack content validity. Also the method of measurement should be appropriate to evaluate the progress of the student in the particular skill. If the student's skill in communicating with a patient is to be evaluated, it could best be done by direct observation rather than a written test. If an inappropriate test is used, the results will lack validity.

Reliability of Evaluation Measures

The reliability of criterion-referenced tests can be assured by careful test preparation. First, we must obtain content validity; second, use a large number of representative test items for each learning outcome or competency. It is well to note that reliable tests may not always be valid. When we say a test is "reliable," we mean it is reproducible — it has the same results from one time to the next. A valid test has the quality of reproducibility but has the added quality of testing what should be tested. In other words, if a test gives the same results time after time, it would be consistent, reproducible, and therefore reliable. But it might be reporting the wrong results consistently. In this case it would not be a valid test.

Distinct Purposes of Evaluation

Evaluation may be accomplished in different ways. When the major goal of education was to train students to recite from memory, oral recitation was the form used for evaluation. Standardized intelligence tests developed early in the twentieth century (1905) by Alfred Binet and others differentiated normal from retarded children and later included the measurement of intelligence of all children. In this classical model the child was evaluated against some group whether in his own field of interest or in an arbitrarily chosen area.

Assessment in these norm-referenced tests is based on criteria of competence in a subject under scrutiny related to the set of norms drawn from a typical population. It is used mainly to grade students in relation to other students who took the same test, and emphasizes grading and the establishment of a rank order of examinees. For example, the attainment of a score of "A" will be better than "B," and so on, or the attainment of a score of 500 will be better than 450. In norm-referenced evaluation, the examiners will probably have in mind the scores that represent the pass, average, above-average, and excellent performance. Performance is related to performance of the group, and one student's placement depends on the quality of performance, good or poor, of the rest of the group.

On a test in a group of 100 students, James may be in the 75th percentile, or in other words, he surpassed the group in the lower 74.9 per cent of students. In another instance, James' score may be third from the top in the upper quarter of the group. Mary's score may be in the first quarter of the group. This interpretation shows the student's position in the group that participated in the test. However, test performance in this norm-referenced system is in relative terms. Although the group is carefully selected and well defined, representing students on a specific level — national, regional, or state — and there has been careful selection of course content in nursing, psychology, and related areas, the test performance is still reported in relative terms. The score indicates only how high the student's placement was in comparison with those who took the test. It does not tell how much the student has achieved or how well she can perform in a nursing situation.

NORM-REFERENCED AND CRITERION-REFERENCED EVALUATION

Norm-Referenced Evaluation

Norm-referenced evaluation theory and practice has been widely accepted by educators and is currently used in making educational decisions in schools of nursing. Generally, norm-referenced tests provide a measurement approach with a wide range of test scores that allows for computation of statistical measures including validity and reliability. One of the most commonly used norm-referenced tests in nursing is the National League for Nursing Pre-Nursing Test. The examination for licensure to practice nursing is a common experience of practicing professional nurses. The results of the college entrance examinations provide information that is valuable in the placement of students according to their levels of reading ability and performance in basic mathematics necessary in nursing.

Criterion-Referenced Testing and Evaluation

Criterion-referenced evaluation measures progress toward a stated objective. It refers to student performance or achievement on an individual basis. It is an assessment of the student's performance in terms of a specific standard stated in the objective. Criterion-referenced evaluation measures provide information on what the student has learned since preassessment, at the end of a course, unit, or program of instruction. The student serves as the source for evaluating the stated objectives. On examination, the results of these evaluations may show deficiencies in the learning sequence that need correction. For example, the student may find the sequence to be without interest or challenge because of a gap in learning sequence. It is also possible that the learning activities may not be related to natural or current nursing experiences. The information obtained should be valuable in revision of the criteria stated in the objectives.

Either norm-referenced or criterion-referenced evaluation, or a combination of the two, may be used in nursing education. However, the trend today is toward criterion-referenced evaluation. One influencing factor may be that accountability for education in terms of time and money is spreading in nursing education. The student is accountable to the teacher and in turn the teacher is responsible for the student. The teacher is accountable to the administrator of nursing, usually the dean, and the administrator is accountable directly or indirectly to the president of the college or university.

Criterion-referenced evaluation is of specific value in nursing education and particularly in clinical nursing, where the teacher needs to know precisely what learning has occurred. Criterion-referenced evaluation pinpoints responsibility. It implies competency-based teaching and learning. The stated competency included in the behavioral objective becomes the criterion against which the teacher measures the achievement of the student toward her objectives.

Criterion-referenced testing and evaluation involves

1. Planning a permanent record for the student.
2. Establishment of behavioral objectives.
3. Preassessment of the student's abilities.
4. Selection of a measuring device, and grading and interpreting the results.

1. The individual written record for the student shows the results of periodic evaluations and includes a summary of the student's progress toward the attainment of the behavioral objectives. This record should be kept in a special locked file. It should be available to the teacher for student guidance. The student should know the progress she is making and how it is being evaluated.

The teacher should keep a "test" file for specific items, such as the short-answer type, anecdotal notes, multiple-choice questions and answers and revisions. The card system may be found easy to handle. If the teacher's "test" file is kept up to date, it will be valuable in answering student's questions that are related to their specific attainments.

2. Criterion-referenced testing and evaluation requires the establishment of specific instructional behavioral objectives for the

students. It should be noted that the student's objectives are also the teacher's objectives. Although it is the responsibility of the student to achieve the objective, the teacher and student work together toward its attainment. These behavioral objectives or subordinate objectives should be for a delimited area of nursing content, such as that expected to be accomplished by mid-term, or at the end of the course or unit of instruction. This makes it possible to focus on relevant nursing activities.

A balance of learning activities and learning outcomes should be selected from cognitive, affective, and psychomotor domains in learning. Objectives must be clearly formulated in terms of standards of performance and learning outcomes. The student will be evaluated on ability to perform the competency stated in the behavioral objective. The required performance should be natural, that is, it should resemble closely that required in the situation in which the competency will eventually be performed. The objectives should have been communicated to the student for acceptance. They should provide for feedback for each student on his errors and successes. In addition, the learning outcomes should not be limited to those simple learning outcomes such as knowledge of medical terms, on the basic level, but include the more complex learning outcomes, the developmental level of learning outcomes, such as analysis, synthesis, and evaluation in the cognitive domain.

3. Preassessment should reveal the ability of the student to perform the subcompetencies of the required competency indicated in the objective. The purpose of preassessment is to find out how much the student knows about the content to be covered and how much she does not know about it. It should provide a base for instruction that can be used for evaluation of progress toward the behavioral objective and subobjectives. The importance of preassessment of student abilities should be stressed; otherwise, the teacher cannot deal expertly with the attainment of objectives. If the teacher is aware of how much the student already knows about the content included in the attainment of the objectives, she can decide the level on which the objectives should be placed. Preassessment may be based on evaluations of the student's attainment in the preceding unit of instruction. It should include a distribution of evaluations from the cognitive, affective, and psychomotor domains.

4. The proper selection of a device or strategy for measuring and evaluating achievement toward objectives is essential. As we have noted, the purpose of criterion-referenced evaluation is to

measure accurately how well each student has attained the stated behavioral objective. Criterion-referenced tests are absolute measures because the individual's score is interpreted in relationship to a fixed criterion, not the scores of other individuals as in norm-referenced tests. The statement of the behavioral objective includes the criterion or standard used in evaluation. The following is a statement of a behavioral objective: "From a table with many instruments, the learner should be able to select the necessary equipment for the performance of a lumbar puncture. Criterion — correctly identify according to the list in the procedure manual."

The student and the teacher decide on the competency in nursing that the student should acquire. The teacher formulates the objective for the competency. This may appear as an exhaustive procedure, but the teacher may already have behavioral objectives to present for discussion, revision, and acceptance to a small group of students. In this way the behavioral objectives may be revised to meet the needs of the students. These objectives include a description of the behaviors the students have accepted as their objectives. When the students have completed the required unit of instruction, the descriptions of the competencies are used as a guide for measuring performance.

The initial preparation of the behavioral objectives includes an objective for each task and standard (competency) that has been identified. The description of the behavioral objective includes not only a statement of the competency but also describes how it will be evaluated. The teacher plans the evaluation for the competency identified in the objective and determines the conditions under which the evaluation will take place.

CHOOSING EVALUATION DEVICES FOR MEASURING ACHIEVEMENT

Evaluation and the Behavioral Objective

The selection of the evaluation device is the responsibility of the teacher. The teacher needs this information for writing the criterion of the behavioral objective. If the goals are specific and stated in terms of observable behaviors, the decision should be relatively easy. For example, in the following competency, "The student will be able to administer medications without errors," it is clear that student achievement will be measured by observation of individual performance for errors made in the administration of medications. In order to clearly state the behavioral objectives, the teacher must have selected the evaluation device.

Figure 4.1 represents an analysis of some competencies or sub-competencies in nursing according to dominant domain, level of learning to be attained, result of the performance, product or process or both, and types of evaluation devices that may be used to measure achievement toward the attainment of the stated competencies in nursing. The result of the performance — product, process, or both — must be considered to determine the specific evaluation device that is appropriate for the situation in nursing. The product is what the student produces, such as a picture. The process is the procedure the student uses or the thinking required in doing it. The development of some competencies involves both process and product. As an example, "Explain accurately how to determine a person's blood pressure using equipment" involves both process and product. The product is the determined blood pressure and the process involves the procedure of thinking through and making decisions or judgments. Appropriate evaluation devices are suggested for each competency. One or more than one of these devices, norm-referenced or criterion-referenced, may be used to evaluate student progress toward the attainment of the competencies in the behavioral objectives.

Some Measuring Devices

When a teacher has analyzed the competencies according to domain — cognitive, affective, and psychomotor — and identified the levels of learning within the domains as well as the process of the behavior, the next step is to select the measuring device to be used. This determination is made on the basis of the content involved in the competency to be tested. Different types of behaviors call for different types of tests; choosing the correct form is important.

In the selection of the measuring device, when the result of the performance is a product such as knowledge, comprehension, application, analysis, synthesis, or evaluation, in the cognitive domain, written tests such as true-false, matching, multiple-choice, completion, short-answer, or essay, may be used. When the result of the performance is a process, performance tests such as role playing, or observation of actual clinical performance in nursing can be used. Affective behaviors are usually by-products of cognitive and

FIGURE 4.1. Choosing Evaluation Devices for Measuring Achievement

Competencies or Subcompetencies in Nursing Education	Dominant Domain and Level of Learning
1. Use data from different sources to arrive at a decision appropriate to the situation.	Cognitive High Level Evaluation
2. Regularly assemble facts and differentiate between relevant and irrelevant facts.	Cognitive Analysis/Synthesis
3. Compile accurately records and information for the preparation of reports.	Cognitive Application
4. Predict accurately reactions of chemical substances.	Cognitive Evaluation
5. Identify correctly medications according to their common characteristics.	Cognitive Knowledge
6. Perceive correctly the effect on a patient's emotions of an inability to communicate.	Cognitive High Level Analysis/Synthesis Evaluation
7. Accurately read patient's chart for information related to his nursing care.	Cognitive High Level Analysis/Synthesis Evaluation
8. Correctly classify drugs used in the treatment of anaphylactic reactions according to the specificity of action.	Cognitive High Level Analysis/Synthesis Decision Making
9. Effectively explain to his mother the medical condition of a child who is seriously ill.	Affective High Level Internalizing
10. Demonstrate how to give a subcutaneous injection skillfully and accurately.	Cognitive (Psychomotor) High Level Integration
11. Dress in accordance with the policy of the school of nursing and the hospital.	Affective Internalizing High Level
12. Arrive at a conclusion of a specific nursing action, by applying recognized criteria for judging.	Cognitive High Level Evaluation Decision Making
13. Write, correct, clear and complete admission "nursing notes" on a patient who is hemorrhaging.	Cognitive (Psychomotor) High Level Integration
14. Explain accurately how to determine a person's blood pressure. Use equipment.	Cognitive (Psychomotor) High Level Integration
15. Effectively explain to a patient the purpose of insulin administration.	Cognitive High Level Evaluation

Result of Performance

Product	Process	*Evaluation Devices*
	*	Observation of individual performance, clinical experience, or field experience. Evaluation of nursing study.
*	*	Multiple-choice examination, any written essay, nursing-care study.
	*	Observation of individual performance.
*	*	Multiple-choice questions, written tests, matching tests.
	*	Multiple-choice questions, matching items.
	*	Multiple-choice questions, role playing, observation of individual performance in nursing situations, essay questions.
*		Written tests, essay, except matching.
	*	Multiple-choice, individual performance.
*	*	Controlled observation of individual performance (criteria list), role playing.
*	*	Controlled observation of individual performance (criteria list).
*		Controlled observation of individual performance (criteria list).
*	*	Individual performance, controlled observation (criteria list), multiple-choice.
*	*	Controlled observation of individual performance (criteria list).
*	*	Controlled observation of individual performance (criteria list).
*	*	Controlled observation of individual performance (criteria list).

psychomotor behaviors. In this instance, observation of individual performance is the most reliable. Multiple observations are recommended since the outward attitude does not always represent the feelings of the student. In the evaluation of psychomotor behaviors, multiple observations of individual performance is favored.

When the measuring device has been selected, it will then be necessary to decide how the results of the test will be evaluated and graded. Evaluation is qualitative and involves the interpretation of the position of the score attained on a particular scale, which may be in terms of the objectives, indicating the expected attainment of the student. For instance, in domain-referenced grading (see Chapter 10), evaluation will be on the basis of specific criteria as well as the level of objectives to be achieved. Grading an essay may be in terms of a certain number of points assigned to the weighted criteria, or the percentage method may be used to indicate the grade. Grading is quantitative in nature and represents a symbol of the interpretation of the student's attainment. It should be noted that grades are summaries and are only small parts of the information included in evaluation. Explanations of the criteria used as a basis for the assigning of these symbols should accompany the grades.

Essay Questions

Essay questions are appropriate for measuring achievement toward behavioral objectives in nursing that are classified in the higher levels of the cognitive domain — analysis, synthesis, and evaluation. These essay questions should begin with words such as "compare," "explain," and "describe." Words representing merely the recall level of the cognitive domain, such as "list," "state," and "identify," should be avoided. The essay questions should be used in relation to instructional behavioral objectives. The objectives should be established and the essay test written according to the expected learning outcomes related to the achievement of the objectives. When the test is constructed, plans should be made to grade it in terms of the stated objectives. Generally, essay tests take a relatively short time to construct, but they consume more time for grading. For this reason, they are most frequently used for small groups of students.

The reliability and validity of essay tests is considered low. The use of several brief essay questions rather than a few questions that require long answers will provide a better spread of the content of the objectives and increase the reliability and validity of the test. A larger and more representative sample of the content of the objectives should be utilized to increase the validity of the test. Optional essay questions should be avoided since exercising their options the students are not all taking the same test. If this instance should exist, the students would lack comparability and the reliability and validity of the test would be reduced. If the same objectives have been accepted by the group, then the essay test should be the same for all members of the group.

The essay test provides information on the student's ability to engage in critical thinking. It provides an opportunity for the student to organize her thoughts and express them in paragraph form. The essay is the product. It is imperative that the teacher is specific in giving directions so that the student knows the purpose of the essay and detailed subordinate topics. These directions should be guided by the statements of behavioral objectives and the criteria that were established when the clearly stated objectives were accepted by the students at the beginning of the course.

The number of essay questions should be limited so that the student can finish them within the time allotted, and this time limit should not be extended for only some of the students. It is obvious that the same conditions should apply to all students in the group; otherwise reliability will be reduced.

It is often said that it is difficult for teachers to grade essay examinations objectively. This may be so when the teacher is influenced by the student's personality, or if there is overemphasis on the value of any one type of content. The teacher should grade according to the content and criteria that she and the students agreed upon at the beginning of the course or unit of instruction. The use of numbers instead of student names for identification purposes on the examinations may reduce the possibility of subjectivity in grading. The actual grading of essay examinations should be performed in a consistent manner. All the students' answers to a given question should be graded at the same time. For example, all the answers to Question No. 1 should be read and graded before going on to Question No. 2, and so on. If this method of grading is used, the grades will be more likely to be on the same basis.

The evaluation of an essay should be weighed according to the importance of predetermined criteria. Each criterion should be assigned a certain number of points, or a certain percentage, depending on the system of grading used. Some graders reserve a certain number of points for over-all impression of the entire essay examination. These points are in addition to those assigned to the specific parts of the test. The results of the test should be given to the students with an explanation of their errors and successes.

Sample Essay Questions

1. Given a nursing situation where a patient has an anaphylactic reaction, compare correctly the underlying physiologic situation in the anaphylactic reaction with those of a normal patient. Criterion – content of recent lecture on clinical nursing care of patients who have an anaphylactic reaction.

2. Given a nursing situation where a patient has an anaphylactic reaction, *justify* the choice of drugs used in this particular incident by application of accurate knowledge of drugs and expected actions. Criterion – content of recent lecture on clinical nursing care of patients who have an anaphylactic reaction.

3. Given a nursing situation where a patient has an anaphylactic reaction, as a result of the application of accurate research findings on the incidence of anaphylactic reactions, *predict* the future occurrence of anaphylactic reactions in the hospital and in the community. Criterion – justify predictions on statements of accurate research findings.

Fill-in or Completion Test Items

As a measuring device, fill-in items, also called completion items, may be written in either question or completion form. These are some examples: "What is the name of the instrument used to measure blood pressure?" "In first aid, what is the first emergency treatment for a bleeding limb?" "The instrument used to diagnose a heart arrhythmia is called _____." "In the home setting, the specific antidote for lye, when taken by mouth, is _____."

Like the essay question, the completion type must stem from an objective or subordinate objective. With the fill-in or completion type of measuring device, the student provides his own answer. This type of question is useful to measure knowledge of facts or information on the basic level of cognitive learning. It is not suited to measurement for the criterion-referenced application or evaluation levels. The limitation of a one-word or one-phase response makes it almost impossible to evaluate the attainment of behavioral objectives at the analysis, synthesis, or evaluation levels.

In writing fill-in items, words that give clues to the answer in the stem portion of the item must be avoided. Careful phrasing is necessary to avoid giving grammatical clues for the right answer. The item should be stated so that only one answer is correct. Item blanks should be equal in length and placed at the end of the sentence. The number of line segments must not match the number of words or letters in the answer.

Completion-type or fill-in items are easy to score if the answer is limited to a specific single word; if not, the grader may spend time deciding whether or not the answer given is equivalent to the key word or words.

Multiple-Choice Test Items

The multiple-choice form of testing has many advantages and is widely used when an objective type test is desired. This form is useful for measuring learning outcomes at the knowledge, understanding, and application levels. The multiple-choice test is favored because it is possible to include a large sampling of learning outcomes.

The multiple-choice form of test consists of an incomplete sentence or a question, which is referred to as the *stem*. It should present a clearly stated problem. The answer is selected from two or more choices that follow. The possible answers are called *alternatives* and the incorrect word or words are called *distracters* or *decoys*. Their function is to distract the students who have not achieved the learning outcomes being measured by the item. The selection of the correct answer involves discrimination between incorrect answers and correct answers. This form reduces the possibility of using any systematic method of choosing, such as might be done in guessing the correct answer by picking every second answer. Weigand feels that the multiple-choice form "can be used to test objectives at the higher levels of the taxonomy more readily than any other objective form."[1] The reliability and validity of the multiple-choice form test items are generally accepted. However, the construction of multiple-choice items that test the analysis, synthesis, and evaluation levels is time consuming, but it can be done.

[1]James E. Weigand (ed.), *Developing Teacher Competencies* (Englewood Cliffs, N.J.: Prentice-Hall, Inc. 1971), pp. 193–197.

The writing of the distractor is the most important and the most difficult aspect of writing the multiple-choice test items. Here are several helpful guidelines:

1. The stem should fully state the central question.
2. The distracters should be definitely wrong but attractive to some of the students who are not sufficiently informed on the content of the objectives.
3. Whenever possible, the items should be arranged in logical order.
4. Answers should be approximately the same length.
5. The use of words such as "always," "sometimes," and "never," should be avoided.

Sample Multiple-Choice Test Items in Nursing

Objective: After completion of an assignment utilizing the components of the nursing process, the students should be able to regularly assemble facts and differentiate between relevant and irrelevant facts. Criterion — correct identification of components of the nursing process in the appropriate sequence.

Competency

Regularly assemble facts and differentiate between irrelevant and relevant facts

Instructions

Circle the number preceding the components of the nursing process that are arranged in the sequence in which they are used.

Test Items

1. Evaluation, intervention, assessment, planning

2. Intervention, planning, assessment, evaluation

3. Planning, assessment, intervention, evaluation

4. Assessment, planning, intervention, evaluation

Subordinate Objective: After reading the bulletin on Cancer Facts and Figures of the American Cancer Society, the student should be able to correctly identify the most frequent site of cancer in men. Criterion — information from bulletin.

Subcompetency

Correctly identify the most frequent site of cancer in men.

Instructions

Circle the number preceding the most frequent site of cancer in men in the United States.

Test Items

1. Colon
2. Prostate
3. Lung
4. Mouth
5. Kidney

Subordinate Objective and Subcompetency: After reading the bulletin on Cancer Facts and Figures of the American Cancer Society, the student should be able to correctly identify the most frequent sites of cancer in women. Criterion — information from bulletin.

Subcompetency

Correctly identify the most frequent site of cancer in women.

Instructions

Circle the number preceding the most common site of cancer in women in the United States.

Test Items

1. Colon
2. Lung
3. Breast
4. Uterus
5. Ovary

True-False Test Items

The basis of a true-false item test is threefold: a statement of the objective, a statement of the competency that has been taken from the objective, and a test item that may be true or false. The student matches the meaning of the test item with the meaning of the competency. The student decides whether to accept or reject the test item statement by indicating whether it is true or false.

The true-false item test can be used in most subject areas in nursing. A relatively large sampling can be obtained in a short time. However, the true-false form as a measuring device must be used very carefully to avoid its many limitations. Some educators consider it one of the poorer forms of selected-response test items. Moreover, it is thought to encourage teachers to pull out statements from textbooks and lecture notes and thus promote a tendency to memorization on the part of the students. Then, too, it is difficult to select test items that are completely true or completely false. There are few situations in nursing when only two alternatives are possible. The true-false examination tests only recognition and the lowest level of cognitive behavior. Because of this limitation, it is not appropriate to test learning outcomes in nursing situations where competencies should be developed to a level higher than recognition.

Students will guess at answers if they have not decided on the "right" one. This makes it difficult to determine which specific learning outcomes have been learned. In comparison, in the multiple-choice item test, selection of incorrect alternatives gives information that may be used to identify misconceptions held by the students. This information can also be used to revise the testing instrument.

The decision to use the true-false item test will depend on the analysis of the competencies that are to be evaluated to determine the result of the performance, a product or process, and the favored evaluation device.

Here are some guidelines for the use of the true-false item test:

1. Only one idea should be used in each statement.
2. Specific determiners such as "never," "in all cases," "sometimes," "often," "generally," or "usually" should be avoided.
3. False statements should not be made out of true statements.
4. There should be approximately as many true statements as false statements.
5. Both true and false items should be of near equal length.

Sample True-False Test Items

Objective and Subcompetency

After attending a lecture on the management of health care in adolescent diabetes, the student should be able to correctly identify key factors in the daily management of these patients. Criterion—content of lecture.

Competency

Correctly identify key factors in the management of the health care of adolescents with diabetes.

Test Items

Instructions

For each of the following statements, circle the "T" if the statement is true and "F" if the statement is false.

T.   F.   Adolescents whose medical diagnosis is diabetes mellitus can rarely be controlled on oral hypoglycemic agents.

T.   F.   Adolescents whose medical diagnosis is diabetes mellitus tend to have more serious complications than those with adult onset of diabetes.

T.   F.   Adolescents whose medical diagnosis is diabetes mellitus should not engage in vigorous athletic competition.

T.   F.   No sugar should be detected in the urine of an adolescent with "controlled" diabetes mellitus.

T.   F.   When an adolescent with diabetes mellitus refuses to take insulin, it may indicate an attitude of denial of having a chronic disease.

Matching-Test Items

Matching-test items can also be used to measure achievement toward behavioral objectives. They can be used to test recall and recognition in the cognitive domain. One of their advantages is that a relatively large sampling of an area being studied can be obtained without consuming much time.

The test items are usually arranged in two columns. A set of words or statements are arranged on the left-hand side of the page, and a set of words or statements are arranged on the right-hand side of the page. The statements are to be matched with each other. The student may be asked to relate associations, ideas, events and their dates, terms and their definitions, objectives to their functions, scientific information to nursing practices, and many other items that may be parallel, equivalent, or contrasting.

In writing the matching test, the items should be limited in length and number and arranged systematically. There should be more answer options than questions. Otherwise, the correct answer may be determined by using the process of elimination. Having too many items may confuse the student and the test may become time consuming. Using variations in grammar in each item to reduce the possible number of clues to the answer should be avoided.

Directions on how to take the test should be clearly stated and indicate what the student should be looking for on the right-hand side of the page. Like other tests where the student selects the answer, the directions should clearly state whether an answer can be used more than once to a given question. It is important to plan to have the entire test on a single page.

Sample Matching-Test Items

Objective: At the completion of Chapter 10, the student should be able to associate the components of the three domains in learning with their specific category. Criterion — criteria as stated in the chapter.

Subcompetency: Identify the names of the components of the domains of learning with their labels or names.

Sample Matching Items

Directions: In the space provided in Column 1, write the number of the word in Column 2 that is associated with it.

Column 1 — Components of Domains

_____ a. Evaluation

_____ b. Integration

_____ c. Synthesis

_____ d. Internalizing

_____ e. Comprehension

_____ f. Organizing

Column 2 — Domains

1. Affective

2. Psychomotor

3. Cognitive

Nursing Care Study — Outline

The nursing-care study has been commonly used in varying forms in nursing education programs, most frequently as an independent or individual study, while the student is assigned to a specific clinical area for nursing experience. It is a study of the complete nursing care of a particular patient and is concerned with all aspects of patient care that are significant for nursing; that is, preventive, curative, and rehabilitative health measures. This comprehensive assessment of the patient's problems provides an opportunity to apply the methodology of nursing, or nursing process, that is behavioral-objective directed. Such an approach allows for the identification of the nursing process and its inherent nursing actions and behaviors that may be evaluated in the cognitive, affective, or psychomotor domains.

The components of the nursing situation should provide for a wide range of study, for example, from analysis to predictions and their verification by application of research findings. The objective and related subobjectives of the study should be clearly stated, including the competencies or standards. A suggested detailed outline should help the student attain the behaviors described in the objective. The method of evaluation should be presented, following the outline, so that the students will know the criteria that are being used and the device used for evaluation and grading.

The following is an outline for a nursing-care study including the objective, competency, and a sequenced method of analyzing the nursing situation to abstract the information that will help the student progress toward the stated objective and its attainment. A checklist can be used for grading in the cognitive, affective, and psychomotor domains and levels of learning within these domains. In each instance the stated level of learning includes the achievement of the lower levels of learning in the hierarchy of the particular domain. For instance, in the cognitive domain, if the student performs on the application level, it is assumed that the student has knowledge and comprehension of that which is applied.

Suggested Plan or Outline for Nursing-Care Study

Objective: After completion of a clinical assignment, the student should be able to regularly assemble facts and differentiate between relevant and irrelevant facts. Criteria — determined by the instructor in the particular clinical area.

Plan to Attain the Selected Objective

Competency: Regularly *assemble* facts and *differentiate* between relevant and irrelevant facts.

Instructions:

1. Analyze the situation for its component parts and describe the devices, equipment, medications, and other measures used as part of the nursing care of the patient, so as to give a comprehensive and concise mental picture of the situation.

2. Differentiate or separate the parts of the situation as you see them; identify and classify them according to their common properties.

3. Group the parts of the situation on an identifiable basis, arrange in hierarchical order, and label. Explain the rationale for the particular classifications.

4. Interpret the resulting data by identifying the components in the nursing situation with the nursing process utilized, the health care given, and the role of the professional nurse.

5. Extend this situation to include possible complications and implications.

6. Make inferences and predict consequences. Explain predictions and hypotheses in terms of cause and effect. Verify your predictions through application of logical principles and researched facts and knowledge in the sciences including nursing. Apply outcomes to other nursing situations in homes, hospitals, and the community.

7. Suggestions for writing:

    a. Limit number of quotations.

    b. Express ideas and knowledge in your own words.

    c. Limit study to three pages typed, double-spaced.

Observation of Individual Performance

Observation of individual performance has been used extensively in the past in nursing. It still remains one of the best means of measuring the progress of students of nursing, particularly in the clinical nursing area. Individual performance refers to the result of a student's action that is evaluated to see whether she has successfully achieved an objective. For example, if an objective is to discriminate between irrelevant and relevant facts and the student's objective is "to assess a patient's problems on admission," what is evaluated is whether the relevant information has been separated from the irrelevant in the student's performance of admission procedures.

One of the disadvantages of the individual observation is the possibility of subjectivity on the part of the teacher or evaluator. However, if multiple methods of measuring attainment toward objectives, such as multiple-choice items, essay questions, and the like, are used, the student should be protected against bias. Recorded observations by more than one teacher are useful for this reason. Of course, there should be no need to protect the student so long as the evaluators are qualified, truthful, and honest in their evaluations and in recording them.

In observation of individual students, the criteria have been established when the objectives were written. The teacher should know the behavioral objectives, the competencies and sub-competencies that are being evaluated, and whether the learning outcome is going to be a process or a product. The student should be familiar with the type of examination that is being used, such as observation of individual performance in a nursing situation in the hospital, community, or home. The teacher will also need to know the established criteria for the student's performance. A criteria sheet should be used. The student may be given a copy of the criteria sheet preceding the evaluation. The student and teacher should agree in advance on the expected observable behaviors to be exhibited at the time of evaluation. For instance, how will the student exhibit respect for the patient and tolerance for his requests? How will the student inform the patient that an uncomfortable treatment will help him later?

SUMMARY

The effectiveness of evaluation depends on the validity and reliability of the types of measurement used. Evaluation strategies may be either norm-referenced or criterion-referenced. Whichever strategy is used, it must be appropriate to the behavioral objective to be attained and the competency that is to be developed.

Norm-referenced tests provide a measurement approach with a large range of test scores that allow for computation of statistical data that may be used to determine validity and reliability of the test scores. The most commonly used norm-referenced tests in nursing include the National League for Nursing Pre-nursing Test and the examinations for licensure to practice nursing as a professional nurse. In the norm-referenced examinations, the student's achievement on the test is measured in relation to the achievement of other students who took the same test.

Criterion-referenced tests measure whether an individual student's achievement meets a specific standard stated in the behavioral objective. When a unit of instruction is completed, the descriptions of the competencies are used as a guide for measuring the student's achievement. The performance may result in either a product or a process. The product is what the student produces, such as an individual performance. The process is the thinking through of the technique or process used in producing the product. Where behavioral objectives including the statement of the competency are used as the standard of performance, criterion-referenced tests should be used. However, norm-referenced test items may be used if they are written for the objectives and their competencies in nursing. They include test items that require selection of answers, such as in multiple-choice test items, and those that use the provision of the answer by the student, such as the essay. These written tests include multiple-choice, completion, true-false items, the essay, the nursing care study, and other forms of "paper and pencil" tests. In addition to written tests, observation of individual performance may also be used.

Preceding the selection of the appropriate device for measuring achievement toward behavioral objectives, an analysis of the competencies in nursing is necessary. The analysis should include the domains into which the learnings fall — cognitive, affective, and psychomotor, the levels of learning to be achieved within these domains, as well as the results of the performance, either product or process, or both. The selection of the device for measurement will depend on the results of the analysis.

REFERENCES

1. American Cancer Society, *Cancer Facts and Figures.* New York: American Cancer Society, Inc., 1975, pp. 6-8, 35.

2. Bernaby, R., et al., *Behavioral Objectives in Curriculum and Evaluation.* Dubuque, Iowa: Kendal-Hunt, 1970.

3. Bloom, Benjamin S., *Taxonomy of Educational Objectives, Handbook I: Cognitive Domain.* New York: David McKay Co., Inc., 1956.

4. Bloom, B., et al., *Handbook on Formative and Summative Evaluation of Student Learning.* New York: McGraw-Hill Book Company, 1971.

5. Fivars, G., et al., *Nursing Evaluation: The Problems and the Process.* New York: Macmillan Publishing Co., Inc., 1966.

6. Glaser, R., et al., *Proficiency Measurement: Assessing Human Performance, Psychological Principles in System Development.* New York: Holt, Rinehart and Winston, 1962.

7. Gronlund, Norman E., *Measurement and Evaluation in Teaching, Instructor's Manual,* 2nd ed. New York: Macmillan Publishing Co., Inc., 1971.

8. _____, *Stating Behavioral Objectives for Classroom Instruction.* New York: Macmillan Publishing Co., Inc., 1970.

9. _____, *Preparing Criterion-Referenced Tests for Classroom Instruction.* New York: Macmillan Publishing Co., Inc., 1973.

10. _____, *Improving Marking and Reporting in Classroom Instruction.* New York: Macmillan Publishing Co., Inc., 1974.

11. Harbeck, Mary B., "Instructional Objectives in the Affective Domain," *Educational Technology,* Vol. 10, No. 1 (January 1970), pp. 49–52.

12. Kibler, Robert J., et al., *Behavioral Objectives and Instruction.* Boston: Allyn and Bacon, Inc., 1970.

13. Krathwohl, David R., et al., *Taxonomy of Educational Objectives, Handbook II: Affective Domain.* New York: David Mckay Co., Inc., 1964.

14. Mager, Robert, *Developing Attitude Toward Learning.* Belmont, Calif.: Fearon Publishers/Lear Siegler, Inc., 1968.

15. _____, *Goal Analysis.* Belmont, Calif.: Fearon Publishers, 1972.

16. McAshan, H.H., *Writing Behavioral Objectives.* New York: Harper and Row, Publishers, Inc., 1970.

17. McLuhan, Marshall, *Hot and Cold.* New York: Signet Books, 1969.

18. _____, *Understanding Media.* New York: Signet Books, 1969.

19. Paduano, Mary Ann, "Evaluation in the Nursing Laboratory: An Honest Appraisal," *Nursing Outlook,* Vol. 22, No. 11 (November 1974), pp. 702–705.

20. Popham, Estelle, Adele Frisbee Schrag, and Wanda Blockus, *A Teaching-Learning System for Business Education.* New York: Gregg Division, McGraw-Hill Book Company, 1975.

21. Popham, W. James, *Educational Statistics: Use and Interpretation.* New York: Harper and Row, Publishers, Inc., 1967.

22. Sax, Gilbert, *Concept Formation — Encyclopedia of Educational Research,* 4th ed. New York: Macmillan Publishing Co., Inc., 1969, pp. 196–205.

23. Taba, Hilda, et al., *A Teacher Handbook of Elementary Social Studies: An Inductive Approach,* 2nd ed. Reading, Mass.: Addison-Wesley Publishing Co., Inc., 1971.

24. Townsend, Edward, et al., *Using Statistics in Classroom Instruction.* New York: Macmillan Publishing Co., Inc., 1975.

25. Tuckman, Bruce W., "A Four-Domain Taxonomy for Classifying Educational Tasks and Objectives," *Educational Technology,* Vol. 12, No. 12 (December 1972), pp. 36–38.

Chapter Behavioral Objectives

Chapter 5 is designed to provide information regarding behavioral objectives, so that at the end of this chapter the learner will be able to

1. Select a subcompetency from Figure 5.1, and construct correctly a behavioral objective using the four steps. Criteria as stated in this chapter.
2. Write two competencies and identify correctly the dominant domain and level of learning within that domain for each competency. Criteria as stated in Chapter 4.
3. Using the same two competencies from number 2, decide on the performance outcome — product or process — and select an appropriate evaluation device for each competency. Criteria as stated in Chapter 4.
4. Using the same two competencies, decide on an appropriate verb. Criteria as stated in this chapter.
5. Analyze a competency for subcompetencies, sequence the subcompetencies logically, and justify the order of priority in her own words.
6. Explain correctly how achievement toward behavioral objectives is determined. Criteria as stated in this chapter.

CHAPTER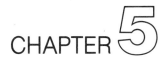

Behavioral Objectives

THE FOUR STEPS IN WRITING BEHAVIORAL OBJECTIVES

When the teacher has analyzed the competencies for dominant and secondary domains and level of learning to be achieved, the result of the performance — product or process — and has decided on the evaluation device to be used, then the next step is to plan to write the behavioral objectives. A behavioral objective is a statement clearly indicating how well a learner must perform an action or behavior under particular conditions.

There are four steps involved in writing behavioral objectives:

1. Determining the actual behavior to be performed in demonstrating the mastery of the objective and selecting the verb to convey the action and the level of the dominant domain.
2. Stating the result of the performance — a product or process — which will be evaluated to determine whether the objective has been achieved.
3. Stating the conditions or situation the learner will be placed under during the time he is performing the behavior being assessed or evaluated.
4. Deciding on the criterion or standard that will be used to evaluate the product or process, or performance.

The Verb as a Key to Writing Behavioral Objectives, Determining the Behavior

Behavior has been described by Mager as an action directly visible or audible, or directly accessible. "An invisible or internal activity can be considered a behavior if it is accessible."[1] The behavioral term expresses the type of activity required of the student. Competencies require different behaviors. There is a difference between the actions of a student who is to "discriminate between information that is confidential and that which is not confidential" and the actions of a student who is to "demonstrate the difference between the position of a patient who has difficulty breathing and one who is breathing normally." The verbs, "discriminate" and "demonstrate" in the previous example convey the behavior to be performed and also denote the level of the dominant domain involved. No competency associated with nursing care of people is dominantly psychomotor. While the nurse performs motor movements as a means to an end, she is actually concentrating on other aspects of the activity. Therefore in these instances, the teacher of nursing works with either the cognitive or the affective domain.

The choice of the verb or action term used to convey an accurate description of the behavior and the level of the dominant domain involved is of utmost importance. The choice of verb is the key to the description of the performance that the learner must exhibit. Action terms should include words or terms that have specific and precise meaning, such as "identify," "describe," "enumerate," "classify," "apply," "categorize." These words may represent any of a wide range of cognitive processes from simple to complex. Words such as "to understand," "to know," "to appreciate," "to enjoy," should be avoided. They are too general, they lack the quality of direction, and do not refer to observable or measureable behaviors. It is important that verbs are selected within the appropriate levels of the cognitive, affective, and psychomotor domains, to provide *continuity* in the evaluation and grading of achievement toward objectives and competencies in the domain-referenced grading scheme (see Chapter 10).

Verbs for Cognitive Competencies

Verbs for cognitive competencies performed in the practice of nursing involve the higher levels of achievement; that is, analysis, synthesis, and evaluation levels. The level of performance, in the cognitive domain selected for students of nursing, should be above

[1]Robert F. Mager, *Preparing Instructional Objectives* (Belmont, Calif.: Fearon Publishers, p.43).

the application level. In selecting the verb, the teacher examines the competency and then classifies it according to domain and level. Figure 5.1 shows examples of competencies, analyzed for domain and level, with selected verbs.

FIGURE 5.1. Competencies Analyzed for Cognitive Domain, Level, and Verb

Competency or Subcompetency	Domain and Level	Verb
1. Correctly select the necessary instruments for the performance of a lumbar puncture.	Cognitive Synthesis	Select
2. Diagnose a nursing situation according to recognized criteria. Accurately reach a conclusion as to the nursing intervention.	Cognitive Evaluation	Diagnose

Figure 5.2 presents a suggested guide for selecting appropriate verbs for competencies at the various levels of the cognitive domain. The cognitive domain includes those competencies and objectives that emphasize intellectual learning outcomes, such as knowledge, synthesis, and evaluation. The six categories in the cognitive domain are arranged in hierarchical order from the simplest behavioral outcomes to the most complex. For example, the cognitive domain begins with knowledge as an outcome and then proceeds through the increasingly more complex levels to comprehension, application, analysis, synthesis, and evaluation. Each category includes behaviors at the lower levels. For example, application includes behaviors at the comprehension and knowledge levels.

Each level of a domain is defined and appropriate verbs are suggested for the different levels in the hierarchy. It is recognized that there is some overlapping in behavioral terms, or verbs, but consistent reference to the definitions of the terms or categories will assist in the selection of the behavioral term or verb that will convey the desired idea in the behavioral objective.

Verbs for Affective Competencies

Achievement of competencies in the affective domain is recognized as important in any profession and of particular importance in nursing. Competencies in the affective domain are concerned with pat-

FIGURE 5.2. Verbs Representing Different Levels of the Cognitive Domain

LOW LEVEL

Knowledge	*Comprehension*	*Application*
Definitions		
Recall and state as it was first perceived.	Grasp meaning of learned material.	Ability to use learned material in new situations.
Verbs		
Recognize	Paraphrase	Translate
Recite	Differentiate	Change
(facts, terms, etc.)	Give an example	Convert
Remember		Use
Name		Apply
List		
Identify		
Tabulate		

terns of adjustment — personal, social, and emotional. Multiple observations of performance are necessary to ascertain if a behavior has become a characteristic of the student. Verbs such as "exhibit" or "demonstrate" are appropriate. When the student consistently exhibits, or willingly demonstrates, the behavior, then it is considered typical or characteristic. It should be noted that cognitive and psychomotor behaviors are usually accompanied by affective behaviors.

For the selection of verbs for affective competencies to be performed, the teacher will examine the competencies and then classify them according to domain and level. See Figure 5.3 for examples.

Figure 5.4 presents a suggested guide for selecting appropriate verbs for competencies at the various levels of the affective domain. The affective domain includes competencies that emphasize feelings and emotion, including interests, attitudes, and appreciations. The affective domain follows the hierarchical pattern of the cognitive domain. The behaviors range over receiving, responding, valuing, organizing, and internalizing, in ascending order of complexity.

		HIGH LEVEL
Analysis	*Synthesis*	*Evaluation*
Ability to identify component parts of learned material.	Ability to create new patterns or structures.	Judge value for given purpose using criteria.
Recognize Divide Analyze Separate Explain	Create Formulate Devise Select Construct Organize Group (elements) Categorize Explain	Compare Contrast Predict Defend Assess Appraise Justify Evaluate Judge Diagnose

FIGURE 5.3. Competencies Analyzed for Affective Domain, Level, and Verb

Competency or Subcompetency	*Domain and Level*	*Verb*
1. Consistently exhibit interpersonal skill while questioning patients to determine their condition and needs.	Affective High Level Internalizing	Consistently exhibit
2. Effectively explain to his mother the medical condition of a child who is seriously ill.	Affective High Level Internalizing	Explain

FIGURE 5.4. Verbs Representing Different Levels of the Affective Domain

LOW LEVEL

Receiving	Responding	Valuing
DEFINITIONS		
Begin to think about attitudes that may be developed. Beginning interest in consideration of rights of patients.	Follow instructions. Do not become involved in activities.	See value of attitud Do not initiate pos action.
VERBS		
Choose	Confirm	Complete
Reply	Help	Differentiate
Ask	Label	Follow
Name	Report	Propose
	Select	Join

Receiving is the lowest level in the scheme and internalizing is on the highest level. Figure 5.4 includes definitions of each of the five categories with appropriate verbs at the different levels in the affective domain. By utilizing the definitions, the teacher will extend the lists of verbs to describe the desired behaviors for the objectives.

Verbs for Psychomotor Competencies

Behavioral objective verbs are selected for the dominant domain of the competency, but it is likely that in the nursing situation the verb selected for the competency of the psychomotor domain will be in either the cognitive or affective domain. Although performance may be automatic, without consciousness being involved, in nursing at the application level of performance and the integration level, consciousness is involved. (See Figures 5.5 and 5.6.) These are stages the learner moves through. It is apparent that the practice of nursing in-

HIGH LEVEL

Organizing	*Internalizing*
Recognize value of behavior and through planning make it possible for others.	Automatic response. Give evidence of consideration and respect for others.
Organize	Perform
Combine	Exhibit
Defend	Demonstrate
Generalize	Act
Integrate	Respect
Relate	
Compare	
Synthesize	

volves consciousness of behavior while using psychomotor skills. The nurse concentrates on what is involved in the performance of each skill. Cognitive learning is essential to the performance of psychomotor skills in nursing and the performance of the skill is a means to an end. For instance, if the competency to be performed is "the accurate administration of medications," the behavior is in the conscious area of the high-level psychomotor domain and it is "integrated" into the nursing situation. Thus the behavior that on the surface is psychomotor, is predominantly in the cognitive domain. In contrast, *skill* is a habit performed spontaneously, without conscious thought. Verbs selected for skills are at the lowest level, such as "lift" or "strike."

For the selection of verbs for psychomotor competencies to be performed, the teacher should examine the competencies and then classify them according to dominant domain and level. See Figure 5.6 for help in choosing an appropriate verb.

FIGURE 5.5. Competencies Analyzed for Psychomotor
Domain, Level, and Verb

Competency or Subcompetency	Domain and Level	Verb
1. Demonstrate how to give a subcutaneous injection skillfully and accurately.	Cognitive and (Psycho-motor) High Level Integration	Demonstrate
2. Write correct, clear, and complete "nursing notes" on a patient who is hemorrhaging.	Cognitive and (Psycho-motor) High Level Integration	Write

The Result of the Performance: Product or Process

Having decided upon the verb that best describes the desired behavior, the next step is to formulate a concise statement of the result of this behavior. The result of the performance of a behavior can be a product, a process, or both. The product can be something as concrete as a painted picture or an essay, or it can be as abstract as a new attitude or communication skill. The process is the physical or intellectual procedure that results in a product.

Conditions of Assessment

The conditions under which the learner will be expected to perform the behavior being assessed could include a description of a given situation in which three patients have been admitted to an emergency room, a situation where the learner will perform certain procedures within twenty minutes, where the student will administer medications while being observed by a supervisor, or given fifteen questions on a special topic to be expected to answer ten of them within twenty minutes, or other variations of the condition.

Criteria for Evaluation

The criteria or standards for the behavioral objective are the standards the student will meet at the completion of the learning experience. These criteria are decided on when the objectives are selected by the student and the teacher, in advance of the performance to be evaluated. There are many sources of criteria. Standard reference sources such as textbooks and journal articles are most commonly used. In the evaluation of a performance in a nursing situation, priority elements would be defined according to the professional experience of the instructor. In the evaluation of psychomotor skills, economy of time, action, and material are important criteria.

The Elements

Five competencies classified according to dominant domain and level of learning are shown in Figure 5.7 with the four components of the behavioral objectives of these competencies. The five competencies and behavioral objectives could be part of a nurse's daily routine. By design, each part of the behavioral objectives has been kept in the same order. Their effectiveness would not be influenced if the order was changed, so long as all of the components of the behavioral objectives are maintained.

SEQUENCING SUBCOMPETENCIES TO ATTAIN BEHAVIORAL OBJECTIVES

Figure 5.8 presents a behavioral objective. "Given a situation in a medical unit in Hospital X, the learner should be able to administer proper medication to a patient with hypertensive heart disease. Criterion determined by the written order on the order sheet and hospital medications manual." In order to attain this objective, certain subcompetencies must be mastered. Furthermore, some of these subcompetencies must be mastered in a specific sequence. All of the subcompentencies included in the diagram, and possibly others that are not included, will be necessary for the attainment of the competency "administer proper medication to a patient with hypertensive heart disease."

Figure 5.9 presents a behavioral objective, "Given a situation where three patients from a street accident are admitted to an emergency room in Hospital X, the learner should be able to evaluate correctly which patient needs immediate medical attention. Criteria determined by clinical instructor." This objective and its

FIGURE 5.6. Verbs Representing the Different Levels of the Psychomotor Domain

LOW LEVEL		HIGH LEVEL
Acquisition	*Application*	*Integration*

DEFINITIONS

Reacting: Think about initiating an action and its elements — start, finish, follow through.

Modifying: Imitate the action while adjusting the position and movements to fit the pattern desired.

Coordinating: Practice the act until smooth patterns of motion are attained.

Habituating: Perform the act automatically with precision and speed without involvement of consciousness.

Anticipating: Perform automatically while experimenting with different patterns of action.

Manipulating: Perform different patterns of motion automatically according to instructions without involvement of consciousness.

Adapting: Perform different patterns of action automatically while consciously dealing with elements of situation.

Integration: Pattern of action becomes a routine part of a whole activity.

VERBS

Perform automatically without involvement of consciousness.

walk	move (self)
swing	reach
swallow	lift
hold	

Perform automatically while consciousness is involved.

coordinate	use	plan
follow	determine	manipulate
demonstrate	measure	write
administer	perform	

competency involve many subcompetencies that utilize high-level achievements in the cognitive, affective, and psychomotor domains, including evaluation, internalization and integration, attained in courses in physiology-circulatory and respiratory systems, psychiatry, and medical-surgical nursing. Such achievements are necessary for successful attainment of the level 4 competency.

PRETESTING AND POSTTESTING — MEASURING THE ATTAINMENT OF BEHAVIORAL OBJECTIVES

Pretesting is used to determine the competencies and sub-competencies the student possesses at the beginning of the unit of instruction or a course. The assessment of the student's achievement will be based on this information. Achievement is defined as the *difference between the competencies and subcompetencies the student has at the beginning of the course or unit, as shown on the pretest, and those that the student has acquired by the end of the instruction period, as shown by the posttest.*

The pretest, of course, must cover the competencies and sub-competencies that it is expected the student will possess at the end of the unit of instruction. In fact, the same test may be used as a pretest and a posttest. For example, the behavioral objectives for this chapter (on page 70) may be used for a pretest and also for a posttest.

If the pretest shows that the student has already acquired the competencies, the time involved in teaching what the student already knows can be spent to achieve more complex and interesting competencies. If the teacher wishes to rewrite the pretest for use as a posttest, the conditions, the behavior, the product, and the criteria must be identical with the original; otherwise it will not be valid and the results will not be accurate.

Pretests provide a base for teaching. Information on prerequisite behaviors sets the stage for implementation of successful instruction. The teacher of nursing needs to examine the results of the pretests and utilize these data related to competencies and subcompetencies to select behavioral objectives and plan learning activities for individual students and groups of students. Individual needs of students may be met by the use of individually paced learning or individually prescribed learning programs that provide a flexible time schedule to achieve the regular behavioral objectives (see Chapter 6).

FIGURE 5.7. Transformation of Competencies into Behavioral Objectives

Competency	Dominant Domain and Level	Verb	Result of Performance Product – Process
1. Correctly select the necessary instruments for the performance of a lumbar puncture.	Cognitive Analysis/Synthesis	Select	Product – Instrument for lumbar puncture.
2. Correctly match the names of drugs with the medical conditions with which they are associated.	Cognitive Analysis/Synthesis	Match	Product – Names of drugs matched with medical conditions with which they are associated.
3. Correctly identify elements of Patient's Bill of Rights within hospital regulations.	Cognitive Evaluation	Identify (decide upon)	Product – Four rights of patients from the Patient's Bill of Rights correctly identified with four comparable hosp regulations that apply to a patient who is goi to have a hysterectom
4. Correctly identify rights of patients from the Patient's Bill of Rights with hospital regulations that are evidence that each right is being pro-tected.	Cognitive Evaluation	Identify (and decide)	Product – Three right of patients from the Patient's Bill of Right identified with three hospital regulations th are evidence that each right is being protecte
5. Consistently exhibit interpersonal skill while questioning patients to deter-mine their condi-tion and needs.	Affective High Level	Exhibit	Process – Interpersor skill while questionin patients.

Conditions of Performance	Criterion	Behavioral Objective
From a table with many different instruments.	According to list in procedure manual.	From a table with many different instruments, the learner should be able to correctly select the necessary instruments for the performance of a lumbar puncture.
Given a list of 10 drugs and a list of medical conditions in two different columns.	Correctly match 8 out of 10 drugs with associated medical conditions.	Given a list of 10 drugs and a list of 15 medical conditions in two different columns, the learner should be able to match the names of the drugs with the names of medical conditions with which they are associated.
Given a situation where a patient is going to have a hysterectomy in a hospital.	Correct identification acceptable to instructor.	Given a situation where a patient is going to have a hysterectomy in a hospital, identify four rights of patients from the Patient's Bill of Rights with four comparable hospital regulations that apply to this patient.
Given a classroom where a teacher is conducting a discussion on the application of the components of the Patient's Bill of Rights to hospital regulations.	Content of the Patient's Bill of Rights and evaluation by the instructor on the domain-referenced checklist.	Given a classroom where a teacher is conducting a discussion on the Patient's Bill of Rights and the application of hospital regulations that are evidence that the patient's rights are being protected, the learner should be able to identify three rights of patients from the Patients Bill of Rights currently incorporated in hospital regulations that are evidence that each right is being protected.
Given a clinic situation where three patients are being admitted.	Determined on domain-referenced checklist — observation of personal performance.	Given a clinic situation where three patients are being admitted, the student should be able to consistently exhibit interpersonal skill while questioning three patients to determine their conditions and needs.

FIGURE 5.8. Sequencing of Subcompetencies

Behavioral Objective: Given a situation in a medical unit in Hospital X, the learner should be able to administer proper medication to a patient with hypertensive heart disease. Criterion determined by the written order on the order sheet and hospital medications manual.

Subcompetency

Apply knowledge of pharmacology of various types of medicines.

Subcompetency

Recall knowledge of methods and dosages of drug administration.

Subcompetency

Recall knowledge of basic anatomy and physiology.

FIGURE 5.9. Division of a Behavioral Objective into Subcompetencies

Behavioral Objective: Given a situation where three patients from a street accident were admitted to an Emergency Room in Hospital X, the learner should be able to EVALUATE correctly which patient needs immediate medical attention. Criteria determined by the clinical instructor.

Subcompetency	*Subcompetency*	*Subcompetency*
Be aware of signs of distress in patients.	Recognize signs of physical deterioration.	Take an accurate history of presenting "complaints".

Subcompetencies

Recall knowledge of mechanisms of anxiety; knowledge of mechanisms of central nervous system; knowledge of mechanisms of circulatory and respiratory systems.

Subcompetencies

Recall knowledge of basic anatomy and physiology; knowledge of basic psychology.

SUMMARY

After the teacher has analyzed the competencies for dominant domain and level of learning to be achieved, has determined the result of the performance, and has decided on the evaluation device to be used, the behavioral objectives may be written. A behavioral objective clearly states how well a learner must perform a behavior under particular conditions. The emphasis is on individual learning.

There are four steps involved in constructing behavioral objectives:

1. Determining the actual behavior and selecting the verb.
2. Determining the result of the performance — product or process.
3. Stating the conditions the learner will be placed under.
4. Deciding on the criterion that will be used to evaluate the product or process.

Competencies and subcompetencies in nursing are identified as the necessary components of behavioral objectives. They are sequenced in hierarchical order, for example, in the cognitive domain, the lowest level represents recall of information, whereas the complex decisions in nursing are dealt with on higher levels.

Pretesting is used to determine the student's status at the beginning of the course or unit of instruction. At the completion of the learning process a posttest is given. The student's achievement will be the difference between the results of the pretest and the results of the posttest. The results of these tests may be used in individual, small-group, or large-group instructional programs.

REFERENCES

1. Bernaby, R., et al., *Behavioral Objectives in Curriculum and Evaluation.* Dubuque, Iowa: Kendal-Hunt, 1970.

2. Corbit, Joan, et al., "A Five-Level Articulated Program," *Nursing Outlook,* Vol. 24, No. 5 (May 1976), pp. 309–313.

3. Dunaway, Jean, "How to Cut Discipline Problems in Half," *Today's Education,* Vol. 63, No. 3 (September–October 1974), pp. 75–77.

4. Glock, Marvin D., *Guiding Learning.* New York: John Wiley & Sons, Inc., 1971.

5. Gronlund, Norman E., *Stating Behavioral Objectives for Classroom Instruction*. New York: Macmillan Publishing Co., Inc., 1970.

6. Guinée, Kathleen K., *Aims and Methods of Nursing Education*. New York: Macmillan Publishing Co., Inc., 1966.

7. Kanfer, Frederick H., "Behavior Modification, An Overview," *The Seventy-second Yearbook of the National Society for the Study of Education,* edited by Carl E. Thorensen. Chicago, Ill.: University of Chicago Press, 1973, pp. 3–40.

8. Kibler, Robert J., et al., *Behavioral Objectives and Instruction*. Boston: Allyn and Bacon, Inc., 1970.

9. Kranovich, Barbara, et al., "The Associate Degree Nursing Faculty and the Resolution on Entry into Professional Practice," *The Journal of the New York State Nurses Association,* Vol. 7, No. 2 (June 1976), pp. 20–22.

10. Levinson, Harry, "Appraisal of What Performance?" *Harvard Business Review.* (July–August 1976), pp. 30–36.

11. Lunsdainc, A., et al., *Teaching Machines and Programmed Learning: A Source Book*. Washington, D.C.: National Education Association, 1960.

12. Mager, Robert F., *Goal Analysis*. Belmont, Calif.: Fearon Publishers, 1972.

13. _____, *Preparing Instructional Objectives*. Belmont, Calif.: Fearon Publishers, 1962.

14. Metcalf, Lawrence E., *Values Education* (41st Yearbook). Washington, D.C.: National Council for the Social Studies, 1971.

15. National Society for the Study of Education, "Behavioral Modification in Education," *The Seventy-second Yearbook of the National Society for the Study of Education,* edited by Carl E. Thorensen. Chicago, Ill.: The University of Chicago Press, 1973.

16. Popham, Estelle, Adele Frisbee Schrag, and Wanda Blockus, *A Teaching-Learning System for Business Education*. New York: Gregg Division, McGraw-Hill Book Co., 1975.

17. Popham, W. James, *Criterion-Referenced Measurement: An Introduction*. Englewood Cliffs, N.J.: Educational Technology Publications, Inc., 1971.

18. Reilly, Dorothy E., *Behavioral Objectives in Nursing Evaluation of Learner Attainment*. New York: Appleton-Century-Crofts, Division of Prentice-Hall, Inc., 1975.

19. Travers, Robert M.W., *Essentials of Learning*. New York: Macmillan Publishing Co., Inc., 1967.

20. Tyler, Ralph, "Behavioral Objectives," *Today's Education,* Vol. 64, No. 2 (March 1975), pp. 41–46.

21. Weigand, James E. (ed.), *Developing Teacher Competencies.* Englewood Cliffs, N.J.: Prentice-Hall, Inc., 1971.

22. Wright, Kenneth B., et al., *Career Education: What It Is and How to Do It.* Salt Lake City, Utah: Olympus Publishing Co., 1972.

Chapter Behavioral Objectives

At the completion of Chapter 6, given the following two competencies:

1. "Work effectively as a member of a team that contributes to effective nursing care of patients."
2. "Effectively handle a difficult child in a hospital unit so the parent leaves the child 'apparently' (from outward appearances) feeling that he is in a secure situation."

The learner should be able to:

1. Classify these two preceding competencies according to dominant domain and level of learning. Criteria as established in Chapter 3.
2. Write a behavioral objective for each of these competencies. Criteria as stated in Chapter 5.

At the completion of Chapter 6, the learner should be able to:

1. Describe correctly the organization of the components of a curriculum according to priorities. Criteria — information in Chapter 6.
2. Explain how balance of learning activities may be achieved in a curriculum. Criteria as stated in Chapter 6.
3. State the six levels of the cognitive domain and supply an appropriate verb for each level. Criteria as stated in figures.
4. Given the terms
   a. "consistent behavior"
   b. "consciousness of performance"
   indicate the dominant domain and level of learning of each of these behaviors. Criteria as stated in Chapter 3 and applied in Chapter 6.

CHAPTER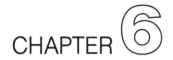

Organization of Materials to Achieve Behavioral Objectives

FORMATION OF A UNIT OF INSTRUCTION, A CURRICULUM

After the faculty has identified and analyzed the competencies and subcompetencies for dominant domain and level of learning to be achieved, decided on the evaluation device, and written a behavioral objective for each competency or subcompetency, then these behavioral objectives are organized into a program, a model, or a unit of instruction such as a curriculum. Just as competencies have subcompetencies, so objectives have subordinate objectives. In education programs, these objectives and subordinate objectives are organized or grouped to accomplish the purpose of the program. They are arranged in a unique hierarchical fashion, in a sequential order so that the attainment of the objectives on each level is a prerequisite to those on the next higher level of accomplishment. Learning experiences, originating from the subject content, and arranged in a sequence of increasing complexity, are planned to help students attain the objectives of the curriculum. Curriculum, then, may be defined as *all the planned student learning outcomes stated in the behavioral objectives.*

The plan for the attainment of the behavioral objectives is projected over the length of time approved by educators and accrediting agencies for colleges and universities and the National League for Nursing as meeting the established patterns for the fulfillment of the requirements for the particular degree, licensure as a professional nurse, or other program. For instance, a curriculum in nursing for a baccalaureate degree may extend over four years. A curriculum for an associate degree in nursing may extend over two academic years, or possibly over two calendar years. This projected overview plan for the entire program or curriculum is divided into years and each year is subdivided into semesters or quarters depending on the pattern established in the university or college. Divisions or subdivisions extend vertically through the semesters or quarters to each course, model or project, and to the individual lesson, the smallest unit of instruction.

The curriculum and each of its units of instruction has its own established objectives stated in behavioral terms. The over-all objectives of the curriculum are stated in more general and inclusive behavioral terms. The statements of behavioral objectives of units of instruction become more specific and easily identified as the units of instruction become smaller, such as a module, a lesson, or a microlesson. The more specific learning outcomes can be accepted as evidence of and contributing to the attainment of the more comprehensive objectives of the larger units of the curriculum. A general objective involves content from many subordinate objectives, ranging from the determination of the patient's blood pressure to making a nursing decision as to when a PRN medication should be given to the patient.

OBJECTIVES OF THE CURRICULUM AND ITS UNITS

The objectives of the curriculum and its divisions should be clearly stated, attainable, and acceptable to the students and the faculty of the program. The objectives should be stated in behavioral terms, so that students will know what is expected of them. It should be noted that statements of the behavioral objectives of the curriculum and its units are translations of the general goals of the program. They are usually observable and measurable forms of behavior. The objectives serve as guidelines and they help focus instruction. A multiplicity of objectives should not be necessary and only those that are significant educationally as learning outcomes, and attainable within time limits, should be included. These objectives should be examined carefully at the beginning of each course and unit of instruction because students' needs change and vary with the prevailing situation in nursing and health. As a part of the curriculum, the objectives are under constant testing by the students and teacher. Particularly in a nursing curriculum, there might be considerable repetition in the learning experiences in the clinical areas unless objectives and their competencies are examined carefully and assigned to students in one specified clinical area. For example, many competencies are common in different areas of nursing and health education, such as "to maintain sterile technique or to maintain medical asepsis," and it is not necessary for students to have the attainment of these competencies repeated. The prevention of repetition in a program is one of the many functions of the curriculum or program committee.

MAINTENANCE OF A "CURRENT" CURRICULUM THROUGH A CURRICULUM COMMITTEE

Purpose and Membership

The content and quality of the curriculum and its learning outcomes are dependent to a high degree on the membership and leadership of the curriculum or program committee. The content of the curriculum in nursing and health education is not static. It changes as the advances in science are applied to nursing care. The task of keeping the education program current, including the learning activities and learning outcomes, is continuous and demanding. This responsibility should be assumed by the curriculum or program committee.

The full membership of the curriculum committee should include representation from all those involved in the education of the learners and the learners themselves, including consumers of health care. They should be kept informed on the pertinent education issues and progress of the program. The purpose of having a working committee is to limit the membership, since otherwise it would be cumbersome as a working unit. Representatives from the student or learner group should be selected or elected by their own groups. Provision for input from these consumers of health education who are trying to achieve the behavioral objectives is necessary. The representatives from the students or other learners should report back to their groups. All the teachers involved in a particular program should participate in the activities of the curriculum committee concerning that program and each teacher should be a member of a subcommittee that represents her special area.

Activities of the Curriculum Committee:

The curriculum committee is made up of subcommittees or subject area committees. The chairperson of the curriculum committee may be chosen or elected by the membership of the committee. The same method of selection of a chairperson may apply to the subcommittees. The dean or head of the program usually attends the first meeting to help orient the committee, to stress the importance of the committee activities and to extend appreciation for participation in the work of the committee. Other activities of a first meeting could include:

1. Definition of the purpose of the committee, which could be "the improvement of learning and instruction in the education program."
2. Election or selection of the chairperson.
3. The chairperson may continue the meeting and arrive at decisions including:
    a. Term of the committee, number and dates of meetings, and time limits for meetings.
    b. Appointment of a recording secretary and provision of an agenda for each meeting.
    c. Provision for circulation of minutes of the meetings.
    d. Appointments and organization of subcommittees.
    e. Schedule for reports from subcommittees.
    f. Agreement on format of reports from subcommittees covering:
       i.   Methods of pretests and presenting results.
       ii.   Statements of behavioral objectives agreed upon by the teachers and students or learners for specific areas including statements of competencies.
       iii. Plans for the evaluation of learner achievement based on pretests.
       iv.   Activities and expected student learning outcomes.
       v.   Tentative plans for acceptance of expected and unexpected learning outcomes.
       vi.   Domain-referenced grading.

Agreement on the format of reports issued by the curriculum and subcommittees is essential; otherwise, at the end of the unit of instruction, a semester, or program, the prerequisite information for a tangible written report to the administrators of the school will not be sufficient or available.

The suggested format of an agenda follows:

AGENDA

A. Roll Call

B. Reading of the Minutes of the Last Meeting

C. Subcommittee Reports

   1. Student Admissions and Evaluation
   2. New Courses
   3. Other

D. Old Business

   1. Arrangements for Pretests for Students
   2. New Data on Need for Curriculum Additions or Omissions
   3. Other

E. New Business

   1. Proposed New Course, Physiology of Illness, Third Semester, 30 Hours
   2. Proposed Merger of Physiology II and Anatomy II, reduced From 60 Hours to 30 Hours
   3. Elements of Physiology and Anatomy Necessary for Medical and Surgical Nursing—How Should This Be Integrated in the Course by the Teacher
   4. Report on Results of Pretests of Freshman Class

F. Summary and Remarks Including a Reminder of the Date of the Next Meeting

G. Motion to Adjourn the Meeting

Teachers, students, and other members of the curriculum committee should be encouraged to become involved in the work of the committee. Each one has a specific contribution to make.

The success of the committee will be influenced by the personality, qualifications, experience, and ability of the chairperson to create a good working environment. The manner in which the members of the committee are greeted by the chairperson and the attitude of the chairperson toward them will influence the cooperation of the committee members. The chairperson may be overanxious about the success of the committee and build up tension and hostility that is felt by the committee members. If a chairperson senses that unfavorable attitudes and stress exist, a reaction memo may help to find out why the committee is not functioning as expected. This inquiry may be put in question form and could consist of only two or three questions and a request for the members NOT to sign their names.

The inquiry could read

What can be done to improve the functioning of the curriculum committee?
What suggestions do you have to be included in the agenda?
Please do NOT sign your name.
Latest return date_____ Thank you,

Chairperson

The chairperson should summarize the results of the inquiry and implement the suggestions, if they are feasible. Follow-up and reporting on the outcomes will be essential. The chairperson usually establishes a routine to:

1. Open and close meetings promptly.
2. Share responsibility for conducting the meetings with other members of the committee as the need arises.
3. Help and guide the members of the committee to clarify their purposes and help them to focus on them.
4. Involve members of the committee in the activities and help them develop their abilities.
5. Delegate responsibility to different members of the committee.
6. Extend appreciation for cooperation and contributions of the members to the success of the committee.

Importance of Varied Representation

The teachers come to the committee meeting with a different perspective from that of the chairperson of the group. Their role has changed from presenting subject content to students, and the process of teaching, to focus on student learning outcomes. They are engrossed in behavioral objectives that the students have accepted as worthwhile pursuing, and learning activities that will produce the best student learning outcomes. These interests may include new courses, merging courses, results of pretests, and helpful ideas from other teachers. The teacher is, no doubt, concerned about the need to conform to a design for reporting the achievement of the students at the completion of the course, semester, or program. While the teacher helps the students achieve their goals, they also need help to attain their own new objectives and the curriculum committee should prove a source of information and help.

The student reflects another perspective. As a representative of the students, she may be concerned about the behavioral objectives, how they are to be attained, and what should be expected when they are attained. Students are concerned about possible changes in the program, such as elements of anatomy and biology necessary for medical and surgical nursing. The feedback from students can acquaint the committee with the effectiveness of the program and what can be done to improve it. The students' reports of their interactions with patients may be so important that the committee may utilize them when they are making revisions in their approaches to bringing health education to the consumer.

The representatives from inpatient, outpatient, and the community population are interested in new knowledge and developments in medical and health care, particularly as it relates to them personally. They look to the professionals for guidance and help in getting this information and related services. They believe that health is now a "right" of the individual. Like the students, these members of the committee are the consumers of health education and they can supply input of great importance to the curriculum committee, and to maintenance of a current curriculum or education program.

If the curriculum committee is responsive to its feedback, which should reflect the situation in nursing and health education, the needs of nursing should be represented and also the needs of the learners. When teachers analyze the current content of a course, topics, concepts, or descriptions of nursing situations for their tasks, set standards, write competencies, and include them in the behavioral objectives, then the curriculum will be kept current.

ORGANIZATION OF LEARNING ACTIVITIES TO ATTAIN BEHAVIORAL OBJECTIVES

Scope, Balance, and Levels of Learning Activities

The scope, balance, and levels of learning activities in the curriculum will be determined by the purpose and behavioral objectives of the education program or curriculum. Learning experiences are activities selected for the purpose of producing learning outcomes. These activities may include listening to a lecture, reading assignments, interviewing a member of a family to determine his health needs, teaching a patient self-administration of insulin, explaining expected actions of medications to a patient in a clinic, or many other activities or experiences in the home, hospital, and community, that help students develop the competencies stated in the behavioral objectives.

Since the objectives of the education program are general, inclusive, and comprehensive, the learning experiences need to be extensive in scope. However, it is not practical to include all the experiences nurses or teachers may encounter in their professional lives, or to include all the relevant knowledge that is now available. But it is necessary to place emphasis on principles and offer guides on how to use new knowledge to help students achieve their future objectives. With this in mind, the scope of learning activities must provide for the development of the learning outcomes stated in the curriculum, as derived from the learning outcomes stated in the behavioral objectives and subordinate objectives.

The design of learning experiences must provide a balance of cognitive, affective, and psychomotor behaviors that contribute to the concept of the health care of the whole person. Since most objectives and their competencies include more than one behavioral domain, the distribution of learning experiences chosen by the teacher should reflect this natural occurrence. Care should be taken to avoid concentration on one category or domain to the exclusion of others. Take for example an objective such as "At the completion of Unit III, pediatric nursing, in a clinic setting, the student should be able to demonstrate how to protect a three-year-old child who is to receive an injection. Criteria as covered in Unit III." This objective involves the cognitive domain as dominant, psychomotor domain as secondary, and the affective domain as the third domain.

Here, the affective domain is of great importance as a learning outcome when working with people, but it must be considered subordinate. This behavioral objective including its competency involves conscious behavior, or thinking about what is being done to protect the child, anticipating possible accidents or complications. All behaviors in the three domains are closely interrelated but as has been mentioned, for measurement and other purposes, it is necessary to select the dominant domain.

Learning experiences or learning activities are arranged in levels of achievement ranging from simple to the more complex. Levels of achievement are based on the degree of complexity of the behavioral objectives. The objectives at each level require the attainment of the behavioral objectives at the preceding levels. This hierarchy of attainments extends upward to the fulfillment of the requirements of the purpose of the program, or in other words, completion of the education program, or graduation from the school. The objectives are stated in behavioral terms indicating what the student is expected to know and what she should be able to do at the different levels of accomplishment.

Sequencing Learning Activities

There are various approaches to arranging learning activities or experiences on levels of learning to assist students in achieving their goals or objectives as efficiently and effectively as possible. For instance, the teacher may ask herself the question "What does the learner need to know as prerequisite behaviors to attain this particular objective?" This question on repetition will produce a sequence of behavioral objectives in the order of the more complex to the least complex. The answers obtained by repeating the same question on successively less complex levels become a sequenced list of behavioral objectives.

Some teachers depend on an order that will evolve as the presentation of learning materials develop. This method may be interspersed by irrelevant remarks and short discussions. "Chatting" in a learning situation is pleasant, but does not always produce the desired learning outcomes. Other teachers use questions from the learners as a method of ordering or sequencing the learning activities, thinking that the learner's needs will be met in this way.

It is agreed that there is no one best method for sequencing learning experiences or activities for the purpose of producing learning outcomes. The learning situation is sometimes unpredictable, just as human behavior is unpredictable and no one single approach will meet the needs of all learners. Success involves interaction, assessment, revising, more interaction, assessment, and revamping to assist students in achieving their objectives as efficiently as possible. Success will even depend on the effectiveness of the teacher in using different methods for sequencing learning activities and the active participation of the students and teacher in planning the activities that the students will choose for the achievement of their own behavioral objectives.

With the change in focus in teaching from teacher process to student learning outcomes, there is need to consider the most efficient and effective ways of sequencing learning activities to attain behavioral objectives. *Sequence* refers to a series having continuity and connection. It is an order of events that follow in succession. *Sequencing of learning activities* refers to efficient planning of activities for the purpose of attaining behavioral objectives. When a method of sequencing activities is used, broad areas of content, situations, concepts, and topics become more manageable in subordinate or smaller parts. Relationships become more evident and lower-level skills can be predicted that should provide a base from which to generate a positive transfer to higher-level skills of attainment. In sequencing learning activities, the focus is on the behavioral objective and its four elements:

1. The actual behavior to be performed in demonstrating the achievement of the objective.
2. The result of the performance.
3. The conditions or situation the learner will be placed under.
4. The criterion or standard that will be used to evaluate the product, or learning outcome.

The teacher and the students should be familiar with some of the different approaches used to sequence learning activities or experiences for the purpose of attaining behavioral objectives. Many educators have contributed to this concept, including Tyler, Bloom and others, Mager, Mager and Beach, Krathwohl and others, Popham, Popham and Baker, Taba, and Gagne.

Gagne's method of sequencing learning activities begins with the simplest types of learning and terminates with problem solving.

Bloom and others have arranged intellectual behaviors into six categories that apply to nursing and health education. Each category is more complex and is dependent on the preceding categories. These categories are (1) knowledge, (2) comprehension, (3) application, (4) analysis, (5) synthesis, and (6) evaluation.

The results of research completed by Taba can also be applied to and utilized in sequencing learning activities in nursing and health education. This research focused on cognitive tasks and teaching strategies needed for the mastery of these tasks. The strategies were arranged in sequential order to bring about behavioral changes in learners. Adaptations of Taba's method of sequencing and Bloom's six categories of intellectual behaviors complement each other.

Taba's method emphasizes the appropriate use of questions. Questions may be used to extend thought on the same level or to make a transition from one level of thought to another level of thought. For example, take the question "What are the elements of the nursing situation when a patient is in shock from apparent bleeding?" In answer to this question, more than one student can give an explanation of his observations. This provides an opportunity for the teacher to explain the nature of the content, clarify the information if necessary, and extend thought on the same level. In making a transition from one level of thought to another level of thought, the first question could be "What are the components of a concept of a patient being discharged from the hospital?" The question on the next level, might be "explain the relationships between the medications ordered by the physician and the expected relief of the patient's symptoms?" A third question could be "what predictions do you make regarding the outcomes of the treatment? Substantiate your predictions with sufficient appropriate scientific information." These are examples of how the focus is changed.

The teacher should be familiar with the different methods and approaches to sequencing used in education that may be used to achieve goals, and then select an approach that is suitable for her specialty and one that she can use comfortably.

Matching Guiding Questions, Tasks, and Intellectual Behaviors

Guiding questions as suggested by Taba are used to abstract tasks on different levels of complexity. In the situation of Mr. Brown, they are matched according to their commonalities with Bloom's six categories of intellectual behavior: knowledge, comprehension, application, analysis, synthesis, and evaluation (see Figure 6.1). The combination of these two methods makes it possible to sequence or order activities according to levels of intellectual behavior from the simple to the more complex. A motion picture sets the scene.

Mr. Brown, a sixty-three-year-old plumber, while driving to work, was hit by an oncoming car. When the ambulance arrived he complained of "a feeling of pressure on his chest." He also had pain in his left arm. He was taken by ambulance to Hospital X and on his arrival in the Emergency Room, was receiving oxygen by mask. Mr. Brown was conscious and anxious about his wife and family and concerned about the notification of his employer. The professional nurse went immediately to his side, introduced herself, and addressed Mr. Brown by name. She asked him "Do you take any medications for diabetes, heart condition, or convulsive seizures?" The nurse assured Mr. Brown that his family and his employer would be notified where he was and about his condition. The nurse then noted Mr. Brown's pulse and respirations. The aide brought the sphygmomanometer and the nurse determined Mr. Brown's blood pressure. She raised the side rails of the bed. She then recorded observations and pertinent findings about Mr. Brown's arrival and condition on his chart. She notified the physician of Mr. Brown's arrival and gave him a summary of the observations and findings. After the physician examined Mr. Brown, he wrote orders for continuation of oxygen by mask, an X-ray of the left upper extremity, a cardiogram, and started an intravenous infusion of 5 per cent dextrose and water.

Analyzing the description of Mr. Brown's situation in Figure 6.1, the first three questions involve the intellectual behaviors — knowledge and comprehension. Many components are enumerated, grouped, and labeled according to their characteristics. These groups could be labeled *oxygen, psychology,* and *sociology.* One of these groups could be labeled specifically for teaching and helping a student achieve an objective such as "At the completion of the unit of instruction, the learner should be able to correctly differentiate (involves analysis and decision making) between acceptable and unacceptable equipment and personnel practices in a patient's unit where oxygen is in use. Criteria based on the content of this lecture."

Guiding questions 4, 5, and 6 resulted in distinguishing the elements that related to the administration of oxygen, giving examples of relationships of identified information, and the formation

FIGURE 6.1. Matching Guiding Questions, Tasks, and Intellectual Behaviors

Guiding Questions	Tasks	Intellectual Behaviors
	1. *Analysis of Data*	
1. Describe the components or elements of Mr. Brown's situation, including equipment.	Enumerate the parts as you saw them.	Knowledge
2. Based on relationships, what parts or elements belong together? Psychology, etc.	Group these parts.	Comprehension
3. How would you identify or label these groups?	Label or categorize	Comprehension
	2. *Interpretation of Data*	
4. Identify what you saw in the motion picture that related specifically to the administration of oxygen to Mr. Brown.	Distinguish or identify the parts or elements of the situation that related to the administration of oxygen.	Application
5. Why were certain precautions taken in the patient's unit?	Give examples and relationships of identified information.	Analysis
6. What significance does this have in the care of a patient who is receiving oxygen therapy?	Form inferences in this patient's situation.	Analysis
	3. *Application of Facts and Principles*	
7. What would happen if certain precautions were absent in this patient's unit? (Physical characteristics of oxygen.)	Predict consequences or potential hazards.	Synthesis
8. Why do you think your predictions would come true?	What are the causal links leading to your predictions or hypothesis, positive or negative? (Justify statements.)	Evaluation (diagnosis.)

of inferences in Mr. Brown's situation. These steps involved the intellectual behaviors of application and analysis. Guiding questions 7 and 8 involve application of facts and principles to predictions or potential hazards in the administration of oxygen, and testing the hypotheses, which involves the process of synthesis and evaluation.

The same description of Mr. Brown's admission to the emergency room Hospital X can be used for helping students achieve an objective related to the psychology of nursing, such as "At the completion of this lecture, the student should be able to analyze correctly a situation in nursing for the psychological reactions of a person to sudden illness or accident, and justify the reactions with principles and facts. Criteria as covered in this lecture."

In implementing the same procedure for helping a student achieve the objective involving the psychological implications of sudden illness for the patient, the teacher may wish to review the components of the same situation, Questions 1, 2, and 3, intellectual behaviors — knowledge and comprehension — and then follow the sequence from that point on to the levels of synthesis and evaluation as shown in studying the administration of oxygen (see Figure 6.2).

Another major component of the situation of Mr. Brown, the sociological implications of sudden illness for the family of the patient, may be used to help the learner achieve another objective. The objective could read "After the study of the situation of Mr. Brown, the learner should be able to evaluate accurately the sociological implications of sudden illness for the patient's family. Criteria as determined in Unit II of instruction." The same order may be used for helping a student achieve this objective. To avoid repetition, the teacher may wish to use the analysis of data, as a review, and then move to the interpretation of data, and lastly to the application of facts and principles where hypotheses are tested and justified with research findings. It should be mentioned that all students do not achieve the highest level of intellectual behavior; however all students should be helped to achieve their greatest potential.

The application and adjustment of the oxygen mask is a nursing procedure of importance in Mr. Brown's situation. The procedure would include an explanation of the purpose of the mask and how the oxygen will benefit Mr. Brown. The physiological implications

FIGURE 6.2.   Two Methods of Sequencing Learning Activities — Guiding
Questions and Intellectual Behaviors

Situation: Mr. Brown's admission to the Emergency Room

Guiding Questions	*Specific for*	*Intellectual Behaviors*
8. Application of principles and	Oxygen Psychology Nursing Procedure Teaching the Family Teaching Mr. Brown Etc.	Evaluation
7. facts.		Synthesis
6. Interpretation 5. of 4. data.		Analysis Application
3. Analysis 2. of 1. situation.	Label Groups Group Parts Describe Components	Comprehension Knowledge
Guiding Questions — Simple to more complex levels		Behaviors — Simple to more complex levels

and also the psychological implications of administration of oxygen
to a member of the family needs explanation, and becomes an essential part of the care of Mr. Brown. The performance of the
psychomotor skill required in the application of the mask and adjustment of the flow of oxygen including the clearing of the nasal
passages and mouth, and the special skin care of the face and eyes,
requires performance like other components of the nursing care of
Mr. Brown, on a level of consciousness and integration on the
highest level into the complete care of Mr. Brown. This procedure
also includes the development of attitudes on the highest level of the
affective domain, which involve *consistent* desirable behavior
toward Mr. Brown, the patient. The behavioral objective that this
experience helps to achieve could read "At the completion of this
unit of instruction the student should be able to demonstrate correctly the application of the oxygen mask and the regulation of the
flow of oxygen to the patient in an emergency situation. Criteria
decided by the teacher."

Some Applications of Organizational Concepts to the Selection of Learning Activities

There is a wide range of learning experiences or activities in nursing and health education. The following suggestions may help to optimize the choices:

1. The behavioral objectives should be examined to determine what the learner should be able to do at the completion of the unit of instruction.
2. The learner's pretest or entry test should be reviewed. Many factors are combined in the learner's behavior at this time. They include the ability to recall, desire to learn, ability to concentrate on the task at hand, and learning pace.
3. The composition of the learning environment and possible interactions between the student and the teacher, patients, or other people should be considered.
4. The level of performance desired should be considered.
5. Only those activities that will provide direct experiences in situations where the current practice of nursing or teaching health will take place and will be available to the learner should be selected.
6. Only those activities that can be performed within the time available should be selected.
7. Only those learning experiences related to the scope or limits of the curriculum content being presented should be selected.
8. Only those learning experiences that provide a balance of the subject content necessary to contribute to the behavioral objectives and purpose of the unit of instruction, that is, cognitive, affective, and psychomotor activities, should be selected.
9. Only those learning activities that provide for the application of factors that influence learning should be selected.

Learning experiences should provide for

1. Subject content necessary to attain the objectives of the students.
2. Opportunities for the learner to achieve the kind of behavior specified in the objective.

3. Activities on the level of the learner's ability (this may be determined by a review of the learner's pretest or preassessment).
4. Activities that relate to the cognitive and psychomotor skills and practice of desirable affective attitudes.
5. Activities that will help learners interrelate theory from social, physical, natural and biological sciences, and the humanities in nursing and health care of individuals.
6. Flexibility in the organization of learning experiences to allow for individual needs of learners and controlled learning situations in nursing practice areas and health education.
7. Opportunities for teachers to observe individual performance of learning activities in various situations.
8. Opportunities for brief intermissions for evaluation of learner achievement.
9. Activities that involve as many senses as possible, including the use of aids.

When cognitive, affective, and psychomotor skills have been decided on, provision should be made for

1. Practice for short periods of time.
2. Practice for the achievement of subcompetencies needed.
3. Practice of skills until effortless performance is achieved.
4. Practice of skills involving consciousness of the situation.
5. Practice of skills accompanied by evaluation and communication with the student or learner.
6. Practice for the next higher level of expansion with the required behavior performed skillfully and consistently with conscious effort.

Utilization of the suggestions for the selection of learning activities should increase efficiency in selecting learning activities and also increase effectiveness of the selected activities.

SUMMARY

After the teacher has analyzed competencies for dominant domain and level of learning to be achieved, has decided on the evaluation device for the product, and written a behavior objective for each competency, the behavioral objectives must then be organized into a curriculum or education program. These objectives are organized around the purpose of the program or unit of instruction in hierarchical fashion so that each level of objectives is prerequisite to those on the next higher level of accomplishments. Learning experiences or activities are arranged to fit in a sequence of increasing complexity established by the behavioral objectives in the program curriculum or other unit of instruction. The emphasis is on the learning outcomes, not on the teacher process. The curriculum or other unit of instruction may be defined as all the planned learning outcomes stated in the behavioral objectives.

The curriculum is broken down into divisions and subdivisions extending vertically to the smallest unit of instruction. Each of these divisions has its own established objectives stated in behavioral terms. The statements of objectives of units of instruction become more specific and more easily identified as the units of instruction become smaller.

The quality of the content of the curriculum is dependent to a high degree on the curriculum committee membership. The curriculum committee membership includes all the teachers, representatives from student groups, and other learner groups, and consumers of health education. Each of these members brings a different perspective to the committee. Each member reports back to his group and receives their reactions. These reactions are relayed to the curriculum committee. The curriculum committee considers the feedback from the different participating groups. If the curriculum committee is sensitive to the needs of consumers of nursing and health education, makes decisions, and implements them in the curriculum, the current needs of nursing and the needs of the learners should be met.

Learning activities or experiences that will provide help for students to achieve the behavioral objectives of the curriculum should be selected by the teachers. These will include experiences broad in scope and sufficient to provide for the development of all the learning outcomes stated in the behavioral objectives in the curriculum. They should be distributed among the cognitive, affective, and psychomotor domains, and on levels ranging from the simple to the more complex or as the content of the objectives indicates. Matching tasks on different levels of complexity according to their commonalities with Bloom's six categories of intellectual behaviors should make it possible to select learning activities that will fit into the sequence established by learning outcomes stated in the behavioral objectives. Examples are shown in Mr. Brown's situation' where learning activities on different levels of complexity are used to help students achieve behavioral objectives related to psychology, sociology, and nursing, on similar levels.

REFERENCES

1. Beland, Irene, et al., *Clinical Nursing — Pathophysiological and Psychological Approaches,* 3rd ed. New York: Macmillan Publishing Co., Inc., 1975.

2. Bernaby, R., et al., *Behavioral Objectives in Curriculum and Evaluation.* Dubuque, Iowa: Kendal-Hunt, 1970.

3. Bevis, E.O., *Curriculum Building in Nursing, A Process.* St. Louis, Mo.: The C.V. Mosby Company, 1973.

4. Bluming, Mildred, et al., *Solving Teaching Problems.* Pacific Palisades, Calif.: Goodyear Publishing Co., 1973.

5. Clark, Cecil, *Using Instructional Objectives in Teaching.* Glenview, Ill.: Scott Foresman and Company, 1972.

6. Crawford, Lucy, *A Competency Approach to Curriculum.* Blacksburg, Va.: Virginia Polytechnic Institute, 1967, Vols. 1–4 (U.S.O.E. Grant No. OEG 6–85–044).

7. Daniel, William A., "Impact of Diabetes on Adolescents," *Texas Medicine,* Vol. 71, No. 11 (November 1975), pp. 56–60.

8. Dececco, John, *The Psychology of Learning and Instruction.* Englewood Cliffs, N.J.: Prentice-Hall, Inc., 1968.

9. Dineen, M.A., "The Open Curriculum: Implications for Further Education," *Nursing Outlook,* Vol. 20, No. 12 (December 1972), p. 770.

10. Dunn, H.L., *High Level Wellness.* Arlington, Va.: Beatty Publications, 1973.

11. Feyercisen, Kathryn, et al., *Supervision and Curriculum Renewal: A Systems Approach.* New York: Appleton-Century-Crofts, 1970.

12. Gagné, Robert M., *Conditions of Learning.* New York: Holt, Rinehart and Winston, 1965.

13. Glasser, William, *Schools Without Failure.* New York: Harper and Row, Publishers, Inc., 1969.

14. Guinée, Kathleen K., *The Aims and Methods of Nursing Education.* New York: Macmillian Publishing Co., Inc., 1966.

15. Hass, Glen, et al., *Curriculum Planning, A New Approach.* Boston: Allyn & Bacon, Inc., 1974, Sections 6 and 7.

16. Howes, Virgil M., *Informal Teaching in the Open Classroom.* New York: Macmillan Publishing Co., Inc., 1974.

17. Jarolimek, John, et al., *Teaching and Learning in the Elementary School.* New York: Macmillan Publishing Co., Inc., 1976.

18. Kanfer, Frederick H., "Behavior-Modification, An Overview," *The Seventy-second Yearbook of the National Society for the Study of Education,* edited by Carl E. Thorensen. Chicago, Ill.: University of Chicago Press, 1973, pp. 3–40.

19. Kemp, Jerrold E., *Instructional Design.* Belmont, Calif.: Fearon Publishers, 1971.

20. Kibler, Robert J., et al., *Behavioral Objectives and Instruction.* Boston: Allyn and Bacon, Inc., 1970.

21. Kinsinger, R.E., "The Core Curriculum for the Health Field," *Nursing Outlook,* Vol. 15, No. 28 (1967), pp. 40–45.

22. Lowenfeld, Viktor, and W. Lambert Brittain, *Creative and Mental Growth,* 6th ed. New York: Macmillan Publishing Co., Inc., 1975.

23. McAshan, H.H., *Writing Behavioral Objectives.* New York: Harper and Row, Publishers, Inc., 1970.

24. McClosky, Mildred C., *Teaching Strategies and Classroom Realities.* Berkeley, Calif.: University of California Press, 1971.

25. Mager, Robert F., *Preparing Instructional Objectives.* Palo Alto, Calif.: Fearon Publishers, 1962.

26. Meehan, M.L., "What About Team Teaching?" *Educational Leadership,* Vol. 30, No. 5 (May 1973), pp. 717–720.

27. National League for Nursing, *Faculty–Curriculum Development, Part VI, Curriculum Revision in Baccalaureate Nursing Education.* New York: National League for Nursing, 1975.

28. National Society for the Study of Education, "Behavioral Modification in Education," *The Seventy-second Yearbook of the National Society for the Study of Education,* edited by Carl E. Thorensen. Chicago, Ill.: The University of Chicago Press, 1973.

29. Popham, Estelle, Adele Frisbee Schrag, and Wanda Blockus, *A Teaching-Learning System for Business Education.* New York: Gregg Division, McGraw-Hill Book Company, 1975.

30. Popham, W. James, et al., *Systematic Instruction.* Englewood Cliffs, N.J.: Prentice-Hall, Inc., 1970.

31. Read, Donald A., et al., *Creative Teaching in Health,* 2nd ed. New York: Macmillan Publishing Co., Inc., 1975.

32. Romey, William D., *Risk-True Love, Learning in a Humane Environment.* Columbus, Ohio: Charles E. Merril Publishing Company, 1972.

33. Sanders, N., *Classroom Questions: What Kinds?* New York: Harper and Row, Publishers, Inc., 1966.

34. Schweer, J.E., *Creative Teaching in Clinical Nursing,* 2nd ed. St. Louis, Mo.: The C.V. Mosby Company, 1972.

35. Shanks, Mary D., et al., *Administration in Nursing.* New York: McGraw-Hill Book Company, 1970.

36. Skinner, B.F., *The Technology of Teaching.* New York: Appleton-Century-Crofts, 1968.

37. Soltis, Jonas F., *An Introduction to the Analysis of Educational Concepts.* Reading, Mass.: Addison-Wesley Publishing Co., Inc., 1968.

38. Stones, E., and S. Morris, *Teaching Practice—Problems and Perspectives.* New York: Harper and Row, Publishers, Inc., 1972.

39. Strasser, Ben B., "Teach for Inquiry. Any Day and Level, Any Subject," *Instructor,* Vol. 82, No. 7 (March 1973), pp. 86–88.

40. Tanner, Daniel, *Using Behavioral Objectives in the Classroom.* New York: Macmillan Publishing Co., Inc., 1972.

41. Thayer, V.T., *Formative Ideas in American Education.* New York: Dodd, Mead & Co., 1970.

42. Tyler, Ralph, *Basic Principles of Curriculum and Instruction.* Chicago, Ill.: University of Chicago Press, 1950.

43. Tyler, Ralph, et al., *Perspectives on Curriculum Evaluation.* Chicago, Ill.: Rand-McNally & Co., 1967.

Chapter Behavioral Objectives

Using information from Chapter 7 as criteria, the learner should be able to
1. Describe correctly how learning takes place.
2. Explain correctly how new concepts may be formed.
3. Differentiate accurately between the traditional role of teacher and student and the role of the teacher and student in criterion-referenced instruction.
4. Describe correctly and in detail the new teacher-learner relationship that has evolved and state the reason.

Given the subcompetency "Explain verbally to a patient so that he understands the difference between abnormal heart symptoms and normal heart functions," decide which factors that influence learning you would apply, and substantiate each in a statement defending its relevance. Criteria as stated in Chapter 7.

Given the subcompetency "Explain what a consumer of health education should know about tetanus," decide which factors that influence learning you would apply, and substantiate each in a statement defending its relevance. Criteria as stated in Chapter 7.

Given the subcompetency "Demonstrate correctly how insulin may be self-administered by syringe," decide which factors that influence learning you would apply, and substantiate each in a statement defending its relevance. Criteria as stated in Chapter 7 and the Nursing Procedure Manual.

Given the subcompetency "Demonstrate ability to communicate with a patient, Mr. Brown, about why he is receiving oxygen by mask," decide which factors that influence learning you would apply, and substantiate each in a statement defending its relevance. Criteria determined by supervisor of nursing care of Mr. Brown.

CHAPTER 7

Understanding the Learning Situation

HOW LEARNING OCCURS — THE PROCESS

Requisites for Learning

Learning is a change in behavior patterns of an individual. It results from an interaction between the individual and a stimulus or a group of stimuli in a situation or environment. There is input from the situation involving one or more of the senses. This input may be simple or something brief, such as a first sight of blood, or as complex as the mental picture or concept of a seriously ill patient in a hospital.

The individual as a learner must be capable of interacting with the stimulus. In the total response of the individual to the stimuli, new behavior patterns are formed, including human reactions. For example, in the learning process an inexperienced student's reaction to a situation where a patient is undergoing kidney dialysis, which requires necessary attachments from a dialyzing machine to the patient's blood vessels, may be one of concern and distraction. Once she understands the benefits to the patient, her view or concept of the whole situation will change. She will see it as a direct help to the patient's physical and mental distress and her feelings and reactions to the dialysis machine and attachments will take on a curative significance.

The Intellectual Environment

The selection and creation of the learning environment that will be suited to the student's background is the responsibility of the teacher. The teacher should be familiar with the student's previous training and experiences, values and attitudes. The intellectual en-

111

vironment should be one that will provide stimuli that will likely be selected by students and lead to their goals or objectives. An exchange of ideas and pleasant student-teacher interaction should exist. For instance, a specific learning situation would not be selected without consideration of the student's level of previous instruction necessary to the formation of desired concepts and attitudes, or learning outcomes. Likewise, a student would not be expected to administer an unfamiliar drug such as an anticoagulant without prior knowledge of the purpose of the administration of the drug, its composition, possible reactions, and the appropriate nursing intervention.

Perception

Learning is a complex process and authorities in education and psychology agree that it is difficult to delineate the precise changes that take place within the individual when experiences are translated into human behavior. However, it is agreed that in the learning situation "a barrier" exists between the conscious and the subconscious mind. Until the stimulus penetrates this barrier, called "the level of awareness," the conscious mind is not involved with the stimulus. The person may see the parts of the situation or the mental image of it, but the conscious mind may not be involved. When the subconscious mind becomes aware or conscious of the stimulus, perception occurs.

Concept Formation

Once the perception stage has been achieved, it is believed that the process of learning progresses to conception. This process involves clarification or decreasing of irrelevant information, with the tendency for the mental picture or "stimulus field" to become integrated. As the process progresses to concept formation, objects or experiences appear singly, or as more than one in relation to others. In this process of association and differentiation, there is no limit to the experiences that are involved; they may include the pleasant or the unpleasant, or those not favorable to positive learning. Thus, when one recalls the concept of an experience, the associated feelings, attitudes, values, and other affective reactions will also be recalled.

Concept formation is the process and the concept is the

product. The concept or mental picture identifies objects, or events, or ideas. These may be concrete, such as an airplane, horse, or ambulance, or abstract, such as happiness, health, or sickness.

There are three basic steps in the formation of concepts:

1. Differentiating the components or elements of objects or events. This involves breaking "wholes" into parts.
2. Grouping components or elements together according to their common characteristics.
3. Naming and labeling groups of components including defining categories related to inclusion or exclusion of new components in the category.

In nursing and health education there is a wealth of experiences that are intense and also natural, that is, not contrived. However, there is a need for teacher guidance to select the right experiences at the right time to attain the desired learning outcomes. When these new experiences are encountered they may not fit into the learner's pattern and she may need to accommodate the "new" by reorganizing or modifying her present pattern. When the learner in nursing is able to internalize the change so that she can utilize the new experience with ease as part of her personal and professional life, she has been able to assimilate the "new" into her pattern.

How to Develop Concepts

One method for identifying concepts is for the teacher to clarify the parameters of a concept through examination of the component parts described in a broad experience. The description may be a presentation of Mr. Brown's admission to the hospital. Or an actual experience can be utilized, such as a visit to an inpatient surgical unit to interview a patient. Consider, for example, a salesman, forty-five years old, who has had his left leg amputated at the knee. He is planning to return home to his wife and a family of two, a boy ten years old and a girl twelve years old. The details of either of these situations or mental pictures of them can be abstracted by first establishing parameters, enumerating the components, organizing them into groups, and labeling them.

A second method for developing concepts is the utilization of questions. A broad experience is presented such as in the preceding instances. After the presentation of the situation, or mental picture, idea, or other experience and a discussion of the topic, the student works in a small group or chooses a partner. They list all questions that occurred to them as they participated in the experience. The questions are sorted and grouped according to common characteristics and appropriately labeled.

Either method will help students to determine specific details that are included in each situation or concept of it. When a category is established, it will be necessary to re-examine the variables within the category so that a general statement can be formulated about the concept.

After the data have been collected and organized, students should be able to develop some relevant generalizations. The generalizing process produces an end product, the concept involving differentiation and synthesis of ideas, situations, and their components or elements.

Transfer of Learning

It is comparatively easy to train people by teaching them what they need to know in a particular situation. But it is not easy to teach people concepts, generalizations, and attitudes that they can utilize in the future to help resolve problems or meet other needs. In the past, many educators believed that the study of certain subjects such as mathematics, or geometry, or science, developed a discipline that was transferable, but psychoeducational research has questioned this theory. Lapp and others concluded that the following three pre-conditions of the student improved the chances of transfer of learning:

1. A broad knowledge of the topic or phenomenon with an awareness of *why* the phenomenon occurs.
2. A positive attitude toward the new situation.
3. A sense of security so that the learner's self-image is protected and the learner may "pause" before reaching a decision.

WHAT AFFECTS THE LEARNING PROCESS

The Teacher

The concept of a teacher of nursing is a nurse who instructs students in schools of nursing, patients, and other learners on nursing and health education. Health education is an integral part of professional nursing practice. The objective to help individuals attain their optimum level of health has not changed. However, with the increasing and expanding need for health education, the degree to which professional nurses and other health professionals participate in health education has increased.

Teaching activities in nursing and health education take place in varied situations, including classrooms and laboratories in colleges and universities where schools of nursing are situated. These activities also take place in inpatient situations in hospitals, outpatient clinics, community agencies, and homes. In nursing care, specifically, the subject content is directed toward the care of the acutely ill patients and their rehabilitation, so that they can adapt and maintain the best possible level of health. The activities have expanded from the prevention of infectious diseases and the teaching of hygiene and safety to knowledge related to preventive medicine and the skills necessary to utilize it in solving health problems.

Preparation of the Teacher

"The extent of the nurses' participation in health education is dependent upon their educational preparation and expertise." (A statement of the American Nurses' Association, Division of Medical-Surgical Nursing Practice and the Division of Community Health Nursing Practice, 1975.)

The professional nurse learns these beginning skills including "assessment of health education needs, planning, and implementing the program and evaluating outcomes of the health education activities" in the generic professional nursing program. For the development, operation, and evaluation of coordinated and integrated health education programs, "additional preparation should include formal courses which are directed toward developing the nurses' knowledge and skills in the following areas:

1. Cultural attitudes and behaviors of people in regard to their health.
2. Theories of roles and role modeling, behavior modification, grief, denial, depression, anger, acceptance, and coping.
3. Dynamics of change.
4. Group and interpersonal communications.
5. Identification and use of community resources.

6. Establishment of relationships with different health professionals.
7. Curriculum development and program methodology.
8. Theories of adult and childhood education.
9. Teaching and learning principles.
10. Implementation of a health education program.
11. Counseling techniques.
12. Use of audiovisual equipment.
13. Program evaluation including process and outcomes."[1]

Qualities of Teachers

The teacher of nursing should meet the qualifications for teachers recommended by the National League for Nursing for their particular specialty. These qualifications include graduation from a baccalaureate program in nursing and the completion of at least a master's program in the nursing specialty in a college or university. Academic preparation in nursing and the sciences, expertise in teaching, and a background of appropriate nursing experience, with well-developed skills in the performance of nursing care are requisites. The teacher of nursing must be prepared for a new role, where the emphasis is on student learning outcomes and the teacher is a director and facilitator of learning.

The student or learner looks to the teacher for guidance and direction and of necessity they spend considerable time together. The teacher and learner should have a partnership relationship. They work together, decide on the behavioral objectives and the expected learning outcomes. The teacher formulates the behavioral objectives. It is the learner's responsibility to achieve the objectives, and it is the teacher's responsibility to help the learner attain them through guidance and the provision of appropriate learning experiences. If the student fails to achieve the objective, the teacher and the student search for the reason and attempt to decide who was responsible, the teacher, the student, or both the student and the teacher.

The teacher must have respect for learning and be able to transmit this respect to students. The teacher needs to be a student as well, since teaching demands knowledge of a wide range of subject content. While teachers do not need to know all the answers, they

[1] American Nurses' Association (Kansas City, Mo.: American Nurses' Association 1975), p. 3.

must be able to guide students to the appropriate reference sources. Usually teachers who possess this interest in learning are flexible and open-minded, qualities essential for effective teaching.

The teacher of nursing and health must be able to organize and utilize learning activities within the learning environment in the classroom, patient unit, clinic, or home. The teacher must have knowledge of modes of teaching, develop them, and use them in the varied teaching situations. The teacher needs to anticipate possible problems, particularly psychological-affective type situations, such as could be experienced in teaching patients or their families. Where the teacher needs to provide psychological support, she must know the subject content and teaching strategies, and these are effective only when the teacher has properly diagnosed the needs of the learners. The teacher must be able to adapt the teaching strategies to the influences on the lesson, such as attitudes of the learners to the subject content or nursing situations. These situations are frequently informal and unstructured and require personal and professional expertise.

Communication skills are a requisite for a teacher of nursing and health. Although human interaction appears simple, there are many times that we are not successful in communicating the real message. If the learner is a patient, he may be more concerned about relief of symptoms than a topic that relates to his future. Weigand recognizes three elements of communication that seem most significant. These are the ability to listen, and respond with empathy, respect, and concreteness. If we know how the other person feels and how he is experiencing the situation (empathy), and if we know our true feelings for this person (respect), and if we listen and respond to the whole message (concreteness), it is probable that the outcome will be more meaningful and productive. Consider for example, a situation in which a student of nursing is corrected for a mistake she has made, by an instructor in a loud voice and in the presence of a patient. The student would be embarrassed and her feelings "hurt." This type of interaction may fail to convey the real message, and carry over undesirable relationships of a serious nature as well.

The teacher must be proficient in group communication skills. These skills are important not only in classroom teaching, but also in teaching outpatient groups and the numerous and varied other situations when nursing and health education are taught. Frequently teachers of nursing are called upon to present materials relative to the health objectives of community organizations.

Teachers must have self-confidence, the ability to meet people and accept them, intellectual curiosity, sincerity, and an appropriate sense of humor. The teacher of nursing needs to have words of encouragement and assurance for students and other learners who are seeking to gain health. Impatience and pessimism rarely improve a learning situation. Basic to these qualifications is good personal physical health, and a healthy self-concept that permits her to use self-assessment. In criterion-referenced teaching, students use self-assessment and the successful teacher must use it also.

Teacher-Learner Relationships

The partnership relationship between two or more persons working together toward a common goal may be accomplished by planned involvement in the undertaking or learning aspects of a lesson. Most approaches to and methods of teaching allow for flexibility and the introduction of the partnership element; some approaches to teaching have a built-in factor that favors the partnership relationship, such as criterion-referenced instruction. As a basic foundation to the partnership relationship, the learner should have a thorough explanation of the structure, content, and objectives of the curriculum or program in which she is studying. The same approach applies to learners in any part of a program. The learner may be a patient, and if so, his curriculum is his health plan. His objectives should be presented in nontechnical language. In this instance, the teacher will, through discussion, be able to determine misconceptions and misunderstandings. Unless the learner · grasps the meaning of his behavioral objectives, his commitment to their attainment will be meaningless. In using the partnership technique, the teacher and the student plan together the different phases of the teaching model, such as restating and revising the behavioral objectives of the clinical experience aspects of the model or unit of instruction. By working together, they close the gap between teacher and learner and improve relationships.

Overcoming the Barriers to Learning Receptivity

Provision of opportunity and time for the learner to reply to relevant information is important. Frequently, the learner is confronted with a "one-way speaker" and without time to respond to his remarks or to ask questions. The teacher may feel relieved that the message was given, and that her responsibility is ended, but the learner may feel frustrated. The learner is sure that something of importance is going on and he feels isolated. The teacher may not return to discuss the message or information and so the confusion in the learner's mind continues to exist.

It is not uncommon for a student to fear loss of prestige with a teacher. A student may think "If I ask that question or give a wrong answer, the teacher may feel I should not be here." Yet even the well-informed professional may not be able to quickly phrase her thoughts. Without feedback, it is unlikely that the teacher can estimate how much the learner knows and without searching questions and discussions the student does not have an opportunity to clarify her thoughts. Discussion would provide the student with an opportunity to analyze and synthesize her thoughts and arrive at more discriminating ideas and decisions. A feeling of difference in status is a common barrier to feedback. This may occur between the teacher and the patient, or in other instances where the person feels that he has inadequate information or lacks the proper vocabulary to convey his ideas. As an example, when a nurse is making "rounds" she may ask a patient a question about his symptoms and he may not be familiar with the terminology she uses. As a result, he may say "Yes, I understand" when he really does not. Rarely will the teacher of nursing return to find out how much the patient really understands. Time limits on personnel and pressing interruptions may prevent short discussions with patients and other learners that would help them clarify their ideas.

In teaching, restrictions on feedback occur particularly in the hospital or other situations where patients are preoccupied with their own illness. It may be that the patient has intense pain or is in an extremely uncomfortable position. Physical discomfort is a very distracting force and until it is relieved a patient will be unable to give his attention, although the information may be very important to him and to his recovery. Of course, the teacher should be sensititive to this type of interference and realize that the patient's one present interest is relief from pain and discomfort. His first concern is to overcome the present pain or ailment, and then his next interest will be, no doubt, "how long will I be in the hospital" or "to what extent will I recover?"

Teachers of nursing occasionally have contact with handicapped patients who are unable to speak. This condition may occur after a laryngectomy or other surgical procedure affecting the throat and voice. The patient may be in the process of learning esophageal speech and will need assurance and help. The teacher will need to provide extra time and special means to communicate, such as a Magic Slate, paper and pencil, checklist of patient needs, or other devices.

Blindness also interferes with communication and feedback unless special aids such as Braille, and increased emphasis on communication through the other senses such as hearing, are utilized. It should be noted that the physically handicapped person may not have as many extraneous distractions as other learners; for instance, the blind cannot see what is happening around them and are frequently more highly interested and motivated to learn about their health than those who are more mobile.

With modern hearing aids and the use of lip reading, communications may be maintained with people who are deaf. However, deafness may remain an obstacle if the teacher does not get the patient's attention before beginning to talk, otherwise he will be unable to establish satisfactory contact and unable to respond to the information presented.

If the teacher and the learner do not speak the same language fluently, a dictionary, language cards, or information shown in both languages are provided in many hospitals, schools, and other agencies. Interpreters may not always be available, and when they are the teacher should always be sure that the proper attitude as well as the message is transmitted accurately. Effective communication including feedback is essential and it is the responsibility of the teacher to see that a communication gap does not exist and that if it should occur, efforts are made to correct the cause.

The communication of ideas or information between persons is an extremely sensitive process and it is easily influenced by the teacher and the learner, or extraneous factors in the environment. A hurried attitude of the teacher, an unkind facial expression, too much noise or too much silence may influence the transfer of thoughts or ideas.

Memories and a series of experiences unfavorable to learning may destroy the possibility of communication. However, the teaching-learning situation is not always solemn. A sense of humor, a newspaper clipping, or remark may help to establish contact and change the attitude of the learner. A short appropriate story and a cheerful teacher may change a poor learning atmosphere to an effective one.

Factors That Influence Learning

The role of the student has come into prominence in the classroom and the teacher of nursing and health has become a director and facilitator. As we have seen, the emphasis has changed from teacher process to student learning outcomes. Although these changes have taken place, the one unchanged area is the teacher's responsibility for consideration of factors that influence learning.

Learning Experiences and Behavioral Objectives

The learner must perceive the learning experience as relevant to an objective. In fact, most single learning experiences contribute to the attainment of more than one objective. The following behavioral objective might be presented to the student: "At the completion of Lesson 6, Unit IV, Medical-Surgical Nursing, the learner should be able to describe the components of the nursing situation of Mr. Smith, who is in a respirator. She should be able to differentiate correctly between the principles of his short-term nursing regimen and the principles of his long-term nursing regimen. Criterion based on Dr. Kelly's lecture and information in the textbook on care of the patient in a respirator." A learning experience that would be relevant to the attainment of this objective would be a visit to a patient who is in a respirator. If the student is "prepared" for this experience, the learning situation will be positive. It must be kept in mind that an initial negative reaction may occur on the part of the student. The student will be seeing, probably for the first time, a helpless patient dependent on a mechanical device for his life. The learning experience will be positive if the teacher has prepared the student before the visit by explaining the purposes of the prescribed medical and nursing care.

Teaching-Learning Environment

As we have seen, change in behavior is brought about by interaction between the individual and a stimulus or stimuli in an environment. The identification of this information is called perception. The more sensitive our perception, the more elements of our experiences can be extracted from the environment. Each individual has different environments. The individual's internal environment is created by past experiences, self-concept, and involves acquired knowledge, attitudes, and skills. The influences from the learner's external environment include the learner's peer group, family membership, socioeconomic status, community, and school, as well as work situations.

In nursing education, an affective environment should be created in which the learner knows that people are more highly valued than procedures. Any practice that contributes to the erosion of the self-image or self-esteem must be open to question. This includes thoughtless remarks by teachers or students about patients and other learners. The student who has a positive self-image will react differently to the same environment than the student whose self-image is negative. The teacher should anticipate situations of this type. The teacher of nursing and health cannot guarantee that learning will take place, but she can establish an environment in which it will most likely take place.

The teaching-learning environment should be structured to provide opportunities to cope with student individual differences. A feeling of easy interaction between the learner and ideas, objects, and patients changes the environment from one that is passive to one that is alive and dynamic. The teacher must be a good listener, imaginative, interested, and flexible to help individual students as members of a group achieve their behavioral objectives in varied environments.

The physical learning environment may be improved by bulletin boards showing materials such as a copy of the Patient's Bill of Rights, displays that carry different relevant messages, pictures of learners teaching patients, and other motivating themes.

Motivation Toward Objectives

Motivation is the process of creating in the individual a need or a desire that prompts action. It occurs when a learner is helped to develop an interest in a specific subject, or delve deeper into a topic.

Motivation can be promoted by convincing the learner of the value of the subject content and the importance of achieving the behavioral objective. Motivation is more likely to occur if students and teachers participate jointly in planning the learning activities and expected learning outcomes that will contribute to their behavioral objectives. The achievement of previous behavioral objectives and competencies also contributes to the student's feeling of accomplishment and supplies a strong motivational influence. With this information the student feels more secure and confident, and studies with a positive attitude. Such accomplishments are valuable and serve as steps or stages of progress toward her next objectives.

The student should be informed of her progress and of how well she is doing during the course of instruction. As an example, when the behavioral objectives and subordinate objectives are sequenced, the subordinate objectives provide planned opportunities to communicate with the student, to inform her of the rate or degree of progress toward the behavioral objectives. The use of self-evaluation checklists also provides opportunities for the student to test herself in order to check her own progress. If the results are positive, they can reinforce continued effort toward the achievement of the objectives. When the learner is motivated, more learning should take place.

Individual Differences

In the learning process, mental responses vary from individual to individual. Individual differences, such as educational background, experiences in the home, church, business, or other places influence these responses. Major interests such as sports, general knowledge acquired through reading, the arts, as well as a complexity of environmental factors result in many different responses for each individual to an identical situation. In addition, the same person may not respond the same way at all times because he may not always interelate facts, emotions, and opinions in the same way.

Because of these many pre-existing influences, students learn at various rates and learning experiences should be designed so that each student will have an opportunity to reach a specified level of mastery or an acceptance level. Bloom's approach adjusts for individual differences by providing "feedback" to the regular instruction and allowing extra learning time for students who need it. Group instruction is supplemented by individual assignments to be completed within reasonable time limits. A variety of alternative resources, such as small-group study sessions, individual tutoring, alternative text-books, are utilized. Criterion-referenced instruction is particularly suited to the needs of individual students.

Association

Association of new behaviors with previously learned behaviors is related to transfer of learning. If the original experience was positive or favorable, the transfer may occur and also the attitude. If the original experience was negative or unfavorable, the student may transfer the attitude to the new learning situation but the transfer will be negative.

Association of behaviors is important in concept formation. Elements or components of situations may be grouped according to their similarities or contrasts. These commonalities provide a basis for grouping components into patterns subsequent to labeling them. When an experience is associated with any other experience the learner has had, it is also differentiated from it.

Active Participation and Practice

Learning is an activity that must be performed by the learner. The teacher directs the student to systematically participate in the learning activities or experiences. It is the teacher's responsibility to arrange the activities or subject content in the best possible sequence to increase the possibilities of learning taking place. In nursing the student must interact with the learning environment where nursing is actually practiced. This is essential if the student is going to develop positive, healthy attitudes. The nursing experiences must be natural, that is, current practice, in a situation where positive relationships exist. The teacher must plan for the active involvement of the student. The student must think about what is being done and actually perform the appropriate skills.

Provision should be made for practice following the initial learning period. The learner should be given an opportunity to evaluate her performance and to present the evaluation to the teacher for suggestions. This procedure is closely associated with success and the learner should be given opportunities to use the newly acquired knowledge and skills in many situations. When factors that influence learning have been understood, exercises for the development of subcompetencies or competencies should be planned for their application.

The Learning Preparation

Learners must have satisfactorily achieved the prerequisite or background learning to respond to the presentation of new learning material. Preassessment should provide the teacher with background information, such as reading ability, learning pace, science grades, and achievement in mathematics. This information should help the teacher of nursing and health to plan for the learner's individual needs, so that her learning proceeds faster and more efficiently.

Sequencing or Ordering Subject Content

As we have seen, materials that are sequenced from the simple to the more complex are more meaningful to the learner than unorganized material. The rate of learning expected is related to the complexity of the content and it is influenced by individual differences. Learning is favored by the presentation of sequenced, short segments of subject content, with opportunities for student participation, practice, and self-evaluation along the way.

Subject content should be organized starting from knowledge and facts, moving to concept formation, principles and eventually to the highest intellectual levels, such as problem solving, predictions, and inferences. Both inductive and deductive methods of treating subject content should be used.

Development of Skills

Jarolimek and Foster define a skill as "a physical activity or intellectual process, or a combination of both, that can be performed in a consistently proficient way in a repeated performance."[1] We usually think of skills as being primarily physical, such as hitting a tennis ball or playing the piano. But there are different types of intellectual skills as well — information processing, interpretation, comprehension, analysis, and synthesis, to name a few. Not all skills involve psychomotor operations. Some skills are entirely intellectual, with no physical or motor involvement. Almost all skills require some degree of cognitive involvement or awareness. Skills do have an affective dimension as well, since the individual likes or dislikes what he is doing. A nursing psychomotor skill may be defined as an activity involving a combination of both cognitive and physical involvement that can be performed in a consistently proficient way in repeated performances. The meaning of the word "proficiency" depends on how well others perform the same act.

---

[1]John Jaroimek, and Clifford Foster, *Teaching and Learning in the Elementary School* (New York: Macmillan Publishing Co., Inc., 1976), p. 249.

The standards and norms of performance are determined by the same performance being observed by a large number of individuals. In evaluating the proficiency of the performance of a skill, the teacher of nursing or health must be familiar with the norms. In addition, the expectations for the level of the student, her age and background, should be considered. When skills are learned well the learner should be able to perform them consistently. This quality of performance will persist provided the individual engages in some amount of maintenance practice. Where a nursing skill is performed inconsistently it usually means that it was not learned initially.

In nursing and health education, each new skill should be presented as an integral part of the whole nursing or health-care situation. For this reason, the skill being taught should not be demonstrated apart from the natural situation or environment in which it will be utilized. In this way the learner should see the usefulness of the skill and come to appreciate those situations when the skill is to be used.

The learner needs to get evaluative information concerning her performance. Positive feedback tells the learner what she is doing and generally it is more productive than negative feedback. It is more predictable in its effect on the individual than negative feedback. To some individuals, negative feedback may act as challenge to do better, but others may be discouraged by it. If this occurs, suggestions on how performance may be improved should follow.

The teacher is still the important influence in feedback, but now some mechanical devices such as teaching machines provide learner feedback. The teacher should keep records on performances, and the student should also have a record of her progress. The learner and the teacher working together can exchange information that may contribute to improvement in performances.

SUMMARY

Learning is a change in behavior pattern of an individual as a result of an interaction between the individual and a stimulus or stimuli in an environment. In the total response of the individual to the stimuli, new behavior patterns, negative or positive, are perceived. The process of learning progresses through association and differentiation to concept formation.

Teachers may assist students to form new concepts by selecting broad experiences or situations, and having them analyze these situations into their elements or components, group these elements, and label these groups. The process must be performed by the learners, otherwise it will lack meaning for them.

The possibilities of transfer of learning are improved when the learner has a general comprehension of the topic, and a knowledge of facts, principles of learning, factors that influence learning, and the ability to apply them.

The teacher of nursing and health must be prepared for her new role of director and facilitator of learning with the emphasis on student learning outcomes. This change in the teacher-learner role increases the need for a partnership relationship. It is the learner's responsibility to achieve the behavioral objective, but it is the responsibility of the teacher to help the student reach the objective.

The teacher of nursing and health needs to have respect for learning and be able to transmit this respect to learners. The teacher should have the ability to organize and utilize learning activities within the learning environment, to apply principles of psychology and education, and she should be proficient in the use of communication skills with individuals and groups. Personal qualifications include self-confidence and intellectual curiosity. Success in teaching nursing and health requires a mix of desirable traits including the ability to use different strategies of teaching. The teacher should possess a healthy self-concept that permits self-reassessment.

In criterion-referenced teaching, the teacher-learner relationship should be on a partnership basis and should be planned. The learner must produce evidence of personal involvement. The teacher has an opportunity to evaluate the progress and success of the students in the attainment of the objectives, to test the validity of the unit of instruction, and to predict processes and learning outcomes.

Although the role of the student has become more prominent, the teacher's responsibility for consideration of the factors that influence learning remains unchanged. Hers is the responsibility for the selection and sequence of the learning experiences and the environment in which they occur, with attention to student motivation and individual background.

REFERENCES

1. Beland, Irene, et al., *Clinical Nursing — Pathophysiological and Psychological Approaches,* 3rd ed. New York: Macmillan Publishing Co., Inc., 1975.

2. Bloom, Benjamin S., *Taxonomy of Educational Objectives. Handbook I, Cognitive Domain.* New York: David McKay Co., Inc., 1956.

3. Bloom, B., et al., *Handbook on Formative and Summative Evaluation of Student Learning.* New York: McGraw-Hill Book Company, 1971.

4. Clark, Cecil, *Using Instructional Objectives in Teaching.* Glenview, Ill.: Scott Foresman and Company, 1972.

5. Davies, Ivor K., *Competency Based Learning: Technology, Management and Design.* New York: McGraw-Hill Book Company, 1973.

6. Dececco, John, *The Psychology of Learning and Instruction.* Englewood Cliffs, N.J.: Prentice-Hall, Inc., 1968.

7. Fivars, G., et al., *Nursing Evaluation: The Problems and the Process.* New York: Macmillan Publishing Co., Inc., 1966.

8. Gagne, Robert M., *Conditions of Learning.* New York: Holt, Rinehart and Winston, 1965.

9. Glock, Marvin D., *Guiding Learning.* New York: John Wiley & Sons, Inc., 1971.

10. Gronlund, Norman E., *Stating Behavioral Objectives for Classroom Instruction.* New York: Macmillan Publishing Co., Inc., 1970.

11. Hass, Glen, et al., *Curriculum Planning, A New Approach.* Boston: Allyn & Bacon, Inc., 1974, Sections 6 and 7.

12. Havighurst, Robert J., *Developmental Tasks and Education,* 3rd ed. New York: David McKay Co., Inc., 1972.

13. Johnson, Lois, et al., *Classroom Management: Theory and Skill Training.* New York: Macmillan Publishing Co., Inc., 1969.

14. Joyce, Bruce, *Models of Teaching.* Englewood Cliffs, N.J.: Prentice-Hall, Inc., 1972.

15. Kanfer, Frederick H., "Behavior-Modification, An Overview." *The Seventy-second Yearbook of the National Society for the Study of Education,* edited by Carl E. Thorensen. Chicago, Ill.: University of Chicago Press, 1973, pp. 3–40.

16. Kemp, Jerrold E., *Instructional Design.* Belmont, Calif.: Fearon Publishers, 1971.

17. Lapp, Diane, et al., *Teaching and Learning: Philosophical, Psychological, Curricular Applications.* New York: Macmillan Publishing Co., Inc., 1975.

18. Levinson, Harry, "Appraisal of What Performance?" *Harvard Business Review,* Vol. 54, No. 4 (July–August, 1976), pp. 30–36.

19. Lifton, Walter M., *Education for Tomorrow, The Role of Media.* New York: John Wiley & Sons, Inc., 1970.

20. Madsen, Clifford K., et al., "You Are Already Using Behavior Modification," *Instructor,* Vol. 81, No. 2 (October 1971), pp. 325–328.

21. McCarthy, Joseph F. (ed.), *The Training of America's Teachers.* New York: Alumni Association of the School of Education, Fordham University, 1975.

22. McClosky, Mildred C., *Teaching Strategies and Classroom Realities.* Berkeley, Calif.: University of California Press, 1971.

23. Mager, Robert F., *Analyzing Performance Problems.* Belmont, Calif.: Fearon Publishers, 1968.

24. _____, *Developing Attitude Toward Learning.* Belmont, Calif.: Fearon Publishers, 1968.

25. _____, *Preparing Instructional Objectives.* Belmont, Calif.: Fearon Publishers, 1962.

26. National League for Nursing, *Faculty–Curriculum Development, Part VI, Curriculum Revision in Baccalaureate Nursing Education.* New York, National League for Nursing, 1975.

27. National Society for the Study of Education, "Behavioral Modification in Education," *The Seventy-second Yearbook of the National Society for the Study of Education,* edited by Carl E. Thorensen. Chicago, Ill.: The University of Chicago Press, 1973.

28. New York State Nurses Association, "An Approach to Teaching Empathy," *The Journal of the New York State Nurses Association,* Vol. 6, No. 3. (November 1975), pp. 10–12.

29. *Nursing Outlook,* "A System for Personalized Instruction," Vol. 24, No. 2 (February 1976), pp. 110–115.

30 Schweer, J.E., *Creative Teaching in Clinical Nursing,* 2nd ed. St. Louis, Mo.: The C.V. Mosby Company, 1972.

31. Shanks, Mary D., et al., *Administration in Nursing.* New York: McGraw-Hill Book Company, 1970.

32. Soltis, Jonas F., *An Introduction to the Analysis of Educational Concepts.* Reading, Mass: Addison-Wesley Publishing Co., Inc., 1968.

33. Silberman, Charles, *Crisis in the Classroom.* New York: Random House, Inc., 1970.

34. Strasser, Ben B., "Teach for Inquiry. Any Day and Level, Any Subject," *Instructor,* Vol. 82, No. 7 (March 1973), pp. 86-88.

35. Sward, Kathleen M., "The Code for Nurses: A Guide for Ethical Practice," *The Journal of the New York State Nurses Association,* Vol. 6, No. 4 (December 1975), Convention Papers.

36. Tanner, Daniel, *Using Behavioral Objectives in the Classroom.* New York: Macmillan Publishing Co., Inc., 1972.

37. Tyler, Ralph W., et al., *Perspectives on Curriculum Evaluation.* Chicago, Ill.: Rand-McNally & Co., 1967.

38. White, Martha Strum, "Psychological Characteristics of the Nurse Practitioner," *Nursing Outlook,* Vol. 23, No. 3 (March 1975), pp. 160–161.

Chapter Behavioral Objectives

At the completion of Chapter 8, the learner should be able to:

1. Select a teaching-learning strategy for the subcompetency "Explain verbally to a patient so that he understands the difference between abnormal heart symptoms and normal heart functions." Decide which factors that influence learning that you would apply and substantiate each in a statement defending its relevance. Criteria as stated in Chapter 7. Defend your decisions in terms of materials presented in Chapter 8.
2. Select a teaching-learning strategy for the subcompetency "Demonstrate how insulin may be self-administered by hypodermic." Decide which factors that influence learning that you would apply and substantiate each in a statement defending its relevance. Criteria as stated in Chapter 7 and the Nursing Procedure Manual. Defend your decisions in terms of using materials presented in Chapter 8.

Using information from Chapter 8 as criteria, the learner should be able to:

1. Describe accurately characteristics of individual students.
2. Describe correctly a strategy that may be used to individualize instruction in large group presentations.
3. Describe correctly how learning activities should be selected for the subcompetency stated in Question 2.
4. Differentiate correctly between the purpose of a regular lesson and a microlesson.

CHAPTER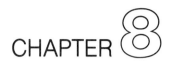

Making Contact with the Individual Learner

THE LEARNER AS AN INDIVIDUAL

Tradition reinforces the idea that teachers teach a class rather than individual learners. However, an audience of one thousand still consists of one thousand individuals. A teacher tries to reach each one. It is only when a teacher begins looking at individual learners that differences among them become apparent.

Individual learners differ in their rates of learning, in their attitudes toward learning, motivation to learn, and even in their interest in the possible learning outcomes.

The challenge is how to make effective contact with the individual learner. Individual learning styles have not been defined; however, it is known that some students profit more from a visual approach, others from a verbal approach, and other students profit more from physical activities. Most students will learn more from a combination or balance of all three approaches.

The teacher must devise methods of teaching or strategies to meet the individual needs of learners in different settings. Focus on individual differences is not new. Fifty years ago the Winnetka Plan and the Dalton Plan were introduced. These plans featured student contracts and individually paced instructional units. The emphasis on this type of strategy has been renewed and more and more programs are introducing adaptations of this approach. There are many reasons for the increased interest, including the spread of criterion-referenced instruction with emphasis on learning outcomes and on accountability for instruction.

INDIVIDUALIZED INSTRUCTION

In planning learning activities to help the student achieve the behavioral objectives, the teacher will need to assess the learner's background, education, aptitudes, abilities, and interests, so as to be able to adjust the components of the program to meet the individual's needs.

Gronlund points out that individualized instruction has often been offered through use of an instructional model with behavioral objectives, self-paced learning materials, and an evaluation system for monitoring and measuring achievement. The characteristics of individualized instructional programs as outlined by Gronlund are

1.   A series of units (or modules) of instruction.
2.   Instructional objectives stated in measureable terms.
3.   Self-paced instructional procedures.
4.   A wide range of instructional materials.
5.   A well-developed testing and evaluation system.
6.   An instructional setting that provides easy access to learning resources.
7.   Flexible time scheduling.
8.   A systematic procedure for managing the program.[1]

The degrees of student freedom of choice of instructional behavioral objectives may be fixed or may be optional. Some programs are set up with predetermined behavioral objectives; in other programs the student selects the behavioral objectives. In either type, the teacher and student must agree on the objectives. In some programs there is a specified time limit, while in others, the student may work at her own pace on each of the divisions of the model or unit of instruction. The student's pretest should provide information to establish the base for the model. The pretest may be used as the posttest.

Some programs are individually prescribed and emphasize a fixed set of behavioral objectives and a specific sequence of learning activities that must be followed for each of the objectives. All students in the group follow the systematic procedure. Each student

[1]Norman E. Gronlund, *Individualizing Classroom Instruction*. New York: Macmillan Publishing Co., Inc., 1974, pp. 21–31.

is placed in a learning sequence determined by individual needs and abilities and students are permitted to complete the prescribed activities at their own pace. The individually prescribed program is flexible and different schools have slightly different approaches and requirements. If a student's pretest shows that she has achieved certain competencies or objectives, adjustments are made in the program that affect the time involved in completing the program.

Large Group Instruction

A large group may consist of twenty-five students in a classroom or two hundred in an auditorium. Large group instruction is frequently used for an introduction to or an overview of a course or unit of instruction; in some instances it may be used for a complete unit of instruction; in some instances it may be used for a complete unit of instruction for a unit. This method avoids duplication of effort and is less time consuming. Because of the large number of students in the group, usually there is not a high degree of feedback. Large group instruction provides an opportunity for small groups to come together and exchange ideas that may be motivating to all the students concerned with the achievement of the behavioral objectives.

Although the group may be large, it is made up of individuals and it can be broken up into small groups and individuals. It is possible to take into account individual differences and to individualize the instruction. The wide range of individual differences among students makes it unlikely that any one method of instruction will meet the varied needs of all students. Some type of adaptation should be used so that more individualized instruction procedures may be utilized and result in better contact with the learner and his needs.

Individualized instruction does not apply to only one method or strategy of teaching. It may range from minor adaptations in group instruction to provision of independent learning experiences. It may be a variation in objectives to be achieved, learning activities, or criteria for evaluation. The teacher can work with each individual even when each one is part of a group. These adaptations and practices are attempts to allow for the individual differences of students and to help learners achieve their behavioral objectives more efficiently. Individualized study does not mean that the learner works alone. It usually takes place in small groups that have been formed from a large group to meet specific needs and interests of learners. The groups are temporary and learners participate in different groups during different class periods. This is no particular procedure except that the class is not taught as a whole group at every meeting. Learners may study the same subject content and may use the same materials in the same sequential order.

The teacher should plan different approaches (lectures, individual study, and so on) to the achievement of the objectives, possibly two or three, and make them available to the learners. The use of a variety of methods and resources might identify the different approaches. In this event, the learners would have a choice that could meet their learning style or mode of learning. Student characteristics will affect their decisions, such as the level at which to start to study a topic or subordinate objective that meets the learner's level of preparation. The teacher can anticipate these levels from the pretest or preassessment of a cumulative record and from consultation with other faculty members and advisors.

A number of specific programs have been described for individualizing instruction, Bloom's Mastery Strategy[2] adjusts for individual differences by producing "feedback" on progress and allowing extra time for the students who need it to achieve the behavioral objectives. The time needed by a student to learn a task is related to the complexity of the task, the preparation of the student, his ability to profit from instruction, perseverance in pursuing the task, and the quality of instruction. The course or subject is divided into units, or natural breaks in the content, such as in chapters. Frequent testing is used to determine learning difficulties, if any, and systematic feedback-corrective procedures are planned. A high level of achievement is stressed for all students. The level of performance is determined by the student's achievement of the standard of mastery, not by comparison of performance with other members of his class.

Keller has described an interesting application of individualized instruction for a large group of students.[3] It was in a course in general psychology offered at Arizona State University, with minor changes, over five semesters with an increasing number of students each semester. In this "at your pace" course, all the course

[2]Norman E. Gronlund. *Individualizing Classroom Instruction.* (New York: Macmillan Publishing Co., 1974), pp. 9–20.

[3]Fred S. Keller, "Good-Bye Teacher," *Journal of Applied Behavior Analysis,* Vol. 1 No. 1 (Spring 1968), pp. 79–89.

requirements could be met in a semester or less.

The course was divided into numbered units, consisting of homework assignments and laboratory exercises. Students took a "readiness" examination at the end of each unit and if they showed mastery of the unit they then moved to the next unit. Lectures and demonstrations in the course were provided when students indicated their "readiness to appreciate them." Examinations were not based on them and attendance at them was not required. These lectures or demonstrations were provided when a certain percentage of the class reached a certain point in the course.

The teaching staff included proctors, assistants, and one instructor. The work in the laboratory was carried out under the direct supervision of a graduate laboratory assistant. A final examination covered all the material in the course. All students registered in the course were required to take the final examination. Credit was given for the number of units completed and the laboratory successfully completed.

Teacher time saved through large group instruction can be used to work with small groups, or for consultation with students in large or small groups, or with students individually on projects. Having large groups may also be more effective in terms of the use of equipment and facilities.

Small Group Instruction

Small groups of students provide opportunities for student interaction and "teacher talk" and "student talk." Because the teacher-learner contacts are more personalized, students often feel more secure in smaller groups, usually six to eight people. Students may be grouped according to similar interests, learning problems, and also abilities. When the objectives are kept in mind in the small group, the students concentrate on their contribution and assume more active roles. Motivation is usually stimulated. The students develop a sense of importance because they listen to one another and share ideas and opinions. They visualize themselves as participants in group effort. They may work together developing sub-competencies in nursing, and when they have completed and reached their objectives, the group disbands and the members may join other groups.

Certain learning activities are best suited to a small group. A formal lecture would be out of place in a small group; in contrast, a discussion would be a "natural." A demonstration by a teacher of a laboratory procedure is best when the learner can see "at first hand."

SELECTION OF LEARNING ACTIVITIES

Planning Learning Activities to Achieve Behavioral Objectives

In planning teaching-learning strategy, the achievement of the behavioral objective is the measure of success. As shown in Chapter 5, there are four steps in formulating a behavioral objective.

1. Determining the actual behavior to be performed in demonstrating the mastery of the objective and the selection of the verb to convey the action and the level of the dominant domain.
2. Stating the result of the performance — a product or process — which will be evaluated to determine whether the objective has been achieved.
3. Stating the conditions or situation the learner will be placed under at the time he is performing the behavior being assessed or evaluated.
4. Deciding on the criterion or standard that will be used to evaluate the product or process, or the performance.

As we know, the verb in the competency is the *key* to the selection of the level of learning to be attained by the learner (see Figures 5.2, 5.3, and 5.4). All learning activities selected should be justified in terms of their contribution toward the promotion of the desired behavior changes, or worthwhile instructional ends, or learning outcomes. Figure 8.1 illustrates the steps that must be completed before the selection of appropriate learning activities.

In this approach, learning activites are selected according to the composition of the competency and to its dominant domain. The dominant domain approach is utilized to highlight the choice of learning activities. If the dominant domain is more cognitive than psychomotor, the learning activity mix will include a predominance of cognitive activities. Figure 8.2, a checklist of learning activities and domains of learning, provides a visual means of checking the balance of cognitive, affective, and psychomotor learning activities, in the one or combination of learning activities that may be choosen for a presentation.

Figure 8.3 shows that although one objective requires one competency for its achievement, each competency will need more than one learning activity for its achievement. Each of the learning activities is developed by presenting material to the student, from the more simple and going to the more complex, that he will wish to participate in, listen to, or read. Although these elements are considered essential to carrying out systematic instruction, they are not sufficient. So that they can be used effectively, it is essential for them to be put together in a coherent way to make it possible to integrate factors that influence learning in the situation. The teacher must organize them to make them more manageable and to make more of an impact on the learners.

The Lecture

The lecture is one of the common ways of organizing learning activities. The lecture is one of the oldest methods of teaching, and it is still used, alone or in combination with other methods of teaching.

Lectures have some advantages; for example, they can be used profitably with learners in almost any subject. A lecture is particularly economical in time. The content of the learning activities can be organized in relation to the behavioral objectives, and a considerable amount of material related to the objectives can be presented in a short time. The lecturer can plan a balance of content that reflects the composition of the three domains, cognitive, affective, and psychomotor, as they occur in the competency. This type of presentation should achieve a reasonable balance of learning activities. However, cognitive learning will dominate.

Affective behaviors may also be taught by this method of presenting learning activities. For example, a lecture involves a particular topic and the lecturer conveys feelings about it in the manner in which it is presented, through his own emphases and gestures. A lecturer can explain different points of view on the same subject and give reports, as part of the content, on recent research. New theories can be interspersed to make the material more current and interesting and at the same time not interfere with the planned sequence of activities.

A lecture can be used effectively with large groups; however, it does have limitations. For example, the opportunity for feedback is limited. Provision for student practice other than note-taking can be planned particularly when a lecture is combined with a discussion.

FIGURE 8.1. Planning Learning Activities to Achieve Behavioral Objectives

Competencies or Subcompetencies in Nursing Education	Dominant Domain and Level of Learning	Result of Performance		Evaluation Devices	Learning Activities
		Product	Process		
1. Use data from different sources to arrive at a decision appropriate to the situation.	Cognitive High Level Evaluation		*	Observation of individual performance, clinical experience, or field experience. Evaluation of nursing-care study.	Focus on behavioral objective for the lesson and participate in clinical nursing or community health experiences. Participate in a field trip. Write a nursing-care study.
2. Regularly assemble facts and differentiate between relevant and irrelevant facts.	Cognitive Analysis/Synthesis	*	*	Multiple-choice examination, written essay, nursing-care study.	Assemble data for report on condition of patients—assemble and differentiate. Report on observations of conditions of three patients.
3. Accurately compile records and information for the preparation of reports.	Cognitive Application		*	Observation of individual performance.	Accurately compile records and information for reports in the pediatric unit. Review reports of pertinent information in the library.
4. Correctly identify medications according to their common characteristics.	Cognitive Knowledge		*	Multiple-choice questions, matching items.	Read on medications and their characteristics in textbook on Pharmacology. Small-group discussion on medications and their characteristics. Review the medication manual on Unit 6. Explanation of special medications and their characteristics to clinic patients.
5. Correctly perceive the effect on a patient's emotions of an inability to communicate.	Cognitive High Level Analysis/Synthesis Evaluation		*	Multiple-choice questions, role playing, observation of individual performance in nursing situations, essay questions.	Observe a patient who is unable to speak. Communicate with a patient by writing when he is unable to speak, and observe his reactions. Explain to a person who is unable to speak why he should take a medication and observe his reactions. Read assignment in Psychology textbook.
6. Accurately read patient's chart for information related to his nursing care.	Cognitive High Level Analysis/Synthesis Evaluation	*		Written tests, essay, except matching.	Read a patient's chart for information on implementation of nursing care. Read special assignment in textbook and give a verbal report in class.

Objective	Domain / Level		Evaluation	Learning Activities
7. Correctly classify drugs used in the treatment of anaphylactic reactions according to the specificity of action.	Cognitive High Level Analysis/Synthesis Decision Making	*	Multiple-choice, individual performance.	Read and study section in textbook assigned by instructor. Listen to lecture on drug therapy, etc. Review physiology notes.
8. Effectively explain to his mother the medical condition of a child who is seriously ill.	Affective High Level Internalizing	*	Controlled observation of individual performance (criteria list), role playing.	Read and study textbooks on nursing pediatrics and psychology. Discuss the child's condition in a small group. Formulate an opinion on the best approach to use.
9. Demonstrate how to give a subcutaneous injection skillfully and accurately.	Cognitive (Psychomotor) High Level Integration	*	Controlled observation of individual performance (criteria list).	Review anatomy and physiology. Assemble the equipment and review the procedure in textbook and treatment manual. Demonstrate the procedure on a mannequin. Administer the subcutaneous injection.
10. Dress in accordance with the policy of the school of nursing and the hospital.	Affective Internalizing High Level	*	Controlled observation of individual performance (criteria list).	Read information on regulations for school. Participate in large group discussions. Participate in small group discussions.
11. Arrive at a conclusion of a specific nursing action by applying recognized criteria for judging.	Cognitive High Level Evaluation Decision Making	*	Individual performance, controlled observation (criteria list), multiple-choice.	Assemble relevant data in the situation. Categorize and label them, synthesize, and evaluate them. Decide upon action based on findings.
12. Explain accurately how to determine a person's blood pressure. Use equipment.	Cognitive (Psychomotor) High Level Integration	*	Controlled observation of individual performance (criteria list).	Read assignment in textbook and procedure manual. Review anatomy involved. Observe the procedure being performed. Assemble equipment for procedure. Practice procedure several times on mannequin. Explain procedure accurately to a classmate.
13. Effectively explain to a patient the purpose of insulin administration.	Cognitive High Level Evaluation	*	Controlled observation of individual performance (criteria list).	Review information on types of insulin used. Discuss use and effect of different types of insulin. Practice explanation to small groups of students.

FIGURE 8.2. Learning Activities and Domains of Learning

Learning Activities	Domains		
	Cognitive	Affective	Psychomotor
1. Lecture	D.D.	Sec.	
2. Guest Lecturer	D.D.	Sec.	
3. Demonstration	D.D.		Sec.
4. Group Discussion	D.D.	Sec.	
5. Field Trip	D.D.	Sec.	
6. Role Playing	Sec.	D.D.	
7. Reading, Writing, Listening, and Speaking	D.D.	Sec.	Sec.
8. Panel	D.D.	Sec.	
9. Questions	D.D.	Sec.	
10. Seminar	D.D.	Sec.	
11. Symposium	D.D.	Sec.	
12. Workshop	D.D.	Sec.	

D.D. = dominant domain
Sec. = secondary domain

FIGURE 8.3. Achievement of a Behavioral Objective and Its Competency

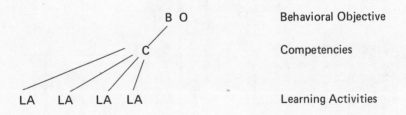

B O   Behavioral Objective

C   Competencies

LA LA LA LA   Learning Activities

Duplicated copies of the lecture are sometimes used and in some schools, attendance at lectures is not required. This regulation presents a challenge to the teacher. However, if the teacher and students plan the objectives together and then the learning activities, they should be anxious to participate, by listening, in the lecture to help achieve their objectives.

Planning the Lecture

If the teacher decides the lecture is the way to present the material relevant to the behavioral objectives, the time should be limited to a thirty- to fifty-minute presentation. The lecturer should make an outline and brief notes on what he is going to say. A list should be made of words and phrases that are associated and pertinent to the material. The plan should have enough detail to keep the speaker from rambling. No one should read a lecture. If they do, they should certainly expect to lose contact with the students.

A series of questions may be used at the beginning of the lecture to be answered at the conclusion of the talk. These questions should be related to the mutual behavioral objectives. The answers may provide an analysis, synthesis, and evaluation of the content included in the presentation in relation to the objectives of the lesson.

Presentation

The presentation of the learning material should be casual rather than very formal. An experienced teacher will use conversational style, in a voice heard throughout the classroom. The delivery should not be too rapid to be understood. Frequently, inexperienced teachers are nervous and speak too fast. If the terminology is new to the students, it should be defined in the lecture.

The teacher should avoid mannerisms. Lecturers should move freely about the classroom and observe what is happening; this is a part of feedback. Some students may be reading a novel, others writing letters, and others daydreaming. If the teacher keeps "eye contact" with the students, it indicates interest.

A lecturer should avoid speech habits such as "okay," "you know." He should use his normal and usual patterns of speech. Teachers should occasionally videotape their presentations and play them back to analyze their speech habits and voice. Sometimes a teacher may be amazed at how he sounds to others.

The Guest Lecturer

A guest lecturer is usually chosen because he or she is an expert in a particular area of the curriculum. This guest may hold an M.D., a Ph.D., an Ed.D., or a masters degree, as well as being an expert in a specific area of the curriculum. A guest lecturer should be introduced to the students with an explanation of his or her background and specialization area. For the purpose of communication, the students should know how to address the lecturer and the type of question that may be related to the lecturer's special field.

The guest lecturer should be given an outline of the behavioral objectives for the lecture and learning activities that could be included, and more specifically, topics, concepts, and situations that were planned for the presentation. The location of the lecture in the series and sequence of learning activities covered by the students and the learning activities to be included in the following lesson should also be given to the lecturer.

The students should have a copy of the behavioral objectives that they and the teacher agreed upon for the lecturer. Each student should know what she needs to get from the lecture to help achieve her behavioral objectives. A preliminary group discussion to identify the students' needs may be held. The lecture could be concluded by a short question-and-answer period. This period of instruction could be conducted by the lecturer or the teacher responsible for the course or unit of it. If the lecture is one of a series, a request could be made of the lecturer to submit suggestions for improvement in the series.

The Demonstration

A demonstration is a visual presentation for the purpose of teaching, using the actual objects, or the actual situation with all of its visible parts. Demonstration is basic to much instruction. It can be used to illustrate and present ideas and learning activities contained in subordinate objectives and objectives in a dramatic way. It is much more interesting to see something happen than to listen to an explanation of it, such as how neutralization occurs when an acid and a base unite. More learning takes place by seeing than by hearing and a demonstration combines both seeing and hearing.

Demonstrations can develop the intellectual skills of the learner. This occurs in biological and physiological science and in nursing and health education. We may recall that the dominant domain of psychomotor skills is cognitive with the affective domain as secondary. The performance of a psychomotor skill involves consciousness. The demonstration provides an opportunity for the learner to speculate on what will happen, how it will happen, and why it will happen. This involves students in applying and practicing skills in the higher levels of cognitive learning, including hypothesizing and predicting.

The demonstration may be performed by the teacher or the learner. The same procedure is followed in either instance. The demonstrator should be sure that he can do what he is supposed to do. To avoid failure, planning is essential. However "spur of the moment" demonstration is usually effective so long as it contributes to the achievement of the behavioral objectives. Poor planning may result in not having the right equipment, such as an extension cord, plug adapter, or other small but essential parts, which will make the difference between success and failure.

The major purpose of the demonstration is to show how something may be done by applying principles or rules to the operation. The teacher is responsible to see that the demonstration is factually and technically correct. The teacher should be able to explain the behavioral objective and how the demonstration relates to it.

For an effective demonstration the teacher

1. Plans to demonstrate so that everyone can see the demonstration.
2. Selects objects that are large enough to be easily seen.
3. Plans to use the opaque projector, overhead projector, or similar apparatus to make small objects visible.
4. Removes unnecessary objects from the situation. What the learner sees will be his concept of it.
5. Selects materials that are available before the group assembles.
6. Plans safety precautions in advance.
7. Plans a summary of the demonstration as part of the whole lesson or learning situation and as contributing to the achievement of the behavioral objective. The demonstration is part of the natural situation and the focus is on the behavioral objective.

The Role of the Learner

The role of the learner is to listen and follow demonstrations carefully and attentively so as to understand the details, and in many instances, be prepared to perform the procedure following the demonstration. The teacher should ask questions to find out whether she is communicating the appropriate ideas. The feedback will help the teacher determine if the learner is ready to practice with limited supervision.

Evaluation will be in terms of the behavioral objective, and specifically in relation to the competency and whether it has been achieved. The observer will note whether important points have been omitted, proper sequence followed, and if future clarification is necessary.

The Presentation of a Patient

It is not always possible for all students to see or talk with a patient who is considered typical for teaching certain nursing procedures. This experience may be made available to all students in a group as part of a lesson, by bringing the patient to the classroom, or the students may visit the patient in his room. The accurate concept of the care of this patient can be improved and clarified through the patient's own description of his condition, and the circumstances that led to his recent illness and admission to the hospital. Students may ask the patient questions related to his present condition and the patient should be allowed to ask questions about his nursing care. A discussion in the classroom should follow, but not in the presence of the patient. The students may have questions they would like to have answered, such as apply to the general appearance of the patient.

Depending on the diagnosis, the student may ask questions related to chemistry, anatomy, psychology, or nursing. The application of subject content makes students appreciate its value in the analysis of the patient's condition.

It may be difficult for a student to remember five symptoms of a patient with congestive heart failure, but she will remember with ease Mr. Smith's discussion when he had congestive heart failure.

Group Discussion

A discussion is an exposition of facts in the conversational mode.

Within the context of teaching it is frequently used and supplemented by the use of anatomical charts, films, drawings, slides, photographs, X-ray films, and the like. The focus of the conversation is the behavioral objective and its subordinate objectives. Groups may be large or small and discussion may be led by the teacher or by a student. This approach is frequently used for planning field trips, group projects, assignments, orientation to community resources, analysis of concepts, formation of new concepts.

It is often claimed that the transmission of information encourages memorization of facts. In using discussion as a teaching strategy, too much teacher-talk and too much explanation should be avoided. Student involvement should be encouraged. Discussion strategy should be appropriately balanced with other strategies in which the teacher guides and facilitates learning.

Involvement in discussion as a strategy of learning

1. Develops students' self reliance.
2. Develops behaviors in the higher levels of cognitive and affective learning.
3. Creates high interest in learning with which the learner identifies.
4. Capitalizes on the social values of learning in the group.
5. Creates an awareness that learning is integrated rather than separated.
6. Encourages the learners' initiative to seek ways of constructing answers to their problems or educational needs.
7. Increases the possibility of the development of favorable attitudes of students toward other students and toward the teacher.
8. Encourages learners to develop fundamental skills and abilities in a meaningful way in the natural situation.
9. Encourages evaluation in terms of behavioral objectives.
10 Encourages self-evaluation.

Teacher-led Discussion

In teacher-led group discussion the content will include the objectives and subordinate objectives of the lesson. The teacher serves as a leader of the group and stimulates and directs active participation of the students.

The teacher

1. Plans a suitable environment for the discussion.
2. Sets a time limit for the discussion.
3. Defines or explains the purpose of the discussion.
4. Prepares questions that range from the simple to the more complex.
5. Focuses the discussion on the objectives.
6. Helps students express or rephrase ideas.
7. Directs questions so that all students are involved in the discussion.
8. Keeps discussion moving to higher levels, for example, application, analysis, synthesis, evaluation.
9. Makes comments that relate to the content of the objectives and that contribute to progress toward achievement.
10. Helps students evaluate different opinions by using data.
11. Makes short summaries at different phases of the discussion.
12. May plan for a discussion to be videotaped for playback and evaluation by the group.

Student-led Discussions

Student-led groups usually evolve from a larger group discussion when the behavioral objectives are complex and there is need for greater active participation with individual contributions. The groups vary in size, usually five to eight students, depending on the size of the large group and the complexity of the behavioral objectives. In student-led groups the teacher does not intervene once the group is established. It is the teacher's responsibility to (1) divide the larger group into smaller groups, (2) break up the groups of students who are friends or who usually work together, (3) have chairs arranged in circles, leaving one chair vacant with each group for an observer, (4) establish a period of five to ten minutes to select a moderator and a recorder/reporter.

The moderator is responsible for (1) stating the purpose of the discussion, (2) dividing time among the speakers and allowing specific time for comments and asking questions, and (3) summarizing the findings of the group. The recorder, after studying her notes and conferring with the moderator, reports briefly to the class. The recorder writes a brief report of the purpose of the discussion and a summary of the outcomes. The recorder should confer with the moderator and have the moderator initial or sign the report.

Buzz Groups

Buzz groups are used after a lecture or a film to increase learner involvement. The teacher asks the large group of students to divide into groups of from four to ten members to discuss the content of the lecture or film, and to select one question they would like to have answered. After discussion, one student reports for each group. A short summary of the group discussion and the question the group would like answered by the teacher is presented.

Groups may be formed in different ways. One method commonly used is to count off the students in groups of three in row one and have them turn around and face three students in row two. Each of these groups selects one question it would like answered. Discussion follows for approximately six minutes and the group formulates an answer to the question. Each group becomes interested in the answer to its own question and also to other questions and answers that the other groups developed. This method provides student involvement and it contributes to cognitive and also affective learning.

Field Trip

A field trip is planned for its contribution to the objectives of the course or project and specifically the behavioral objectives that the teacher and student decided to achieve. Field trips can be used to help students achieve different objectives because of the wealth of information available in a well planned learning visit. A field trip contributes dominantly to the cognitive domain and secondarily to the affective domain. Field trips are extensions of learning experiences, particularly classroom discussions, or possibly a motion picture on a topic that extends into the community.

A student of nursing should be prepared to function effectively in health situations in the community as a professional nurse. This objective involves many subordinate objectives. Observation of socioeconomic, cultural, and other conditions in the community and their effect on the health of the individuals enables the student to develop a "feeling" for people and individuals. Students become aware of the impact of the conditions on nursing and health education and on themselves as individuals and future professionals.

In planning a field trip the teacher should

1.   Contact the administrator of the agency or school to be visited

for permission to bring student observers for a visit.

2. Advise the administrator of the purpose of the visit and the number of students, usually not more than fifteen, to expect.

3. Obtain the name of the agency's representative who will accompany the students and brief them on particular details.

4. Arrange time of arrival and departure of students.

5. Review the behavioral objectives with the students so that they will know the type of observations that will relate to their objectives.

6. Ask each student for a written summary stating behavioral objectives and telling how the field trip contributed to her achievement. This assignment provides one means for the evaluation of the learning experience.

Role Playing

Role playing is a technique and an activity that can be used to help students increase understanding by assuming the roles of participants in a situation. The student becomes involved in the examination of his values and how to negotiate and compromise. Students act and react spontaneously as they interact with one another. These interactions involve ideas, feelings, and attitudes. Such experiences help students become more self-reliant, and to develop affective behaviors.

Role playing a problem situation provides the students with direct examples of human interaction, and they can examine the process at first hand. There may be several solutions to a problem and they can see the impact of their emotions on the solutions that evolve. This experience helps students develop a sensitivity for the feelings of others and relate it to ethical standards.

Role playing offers many opportunities to achieve affective competencies such as "Consistently show respect for the feelings of individual patients." For instance, a student of nursing may conduct an interview on dietary habits with a patient whose understanding of English is limited as well as his understanding of the medical terminology. As a result, the patient asks the same questions repeatedly and the student becomes annoyed. Two students volunteer to play these roles, one the patient and one the student of nursing. The performers present the solutions to the problems at the end of the performance or after a planning or discussion session. The observers develop the criteria for the evaluation of the solution to the problems. Evaluation is one of the high levels of cognitive learning and the criteria should be on that level. They present the criteria to the class and the short discussion that follows involves student suggestions and possibly other solutions. To further the learning outcomes, students may be assigned to interview patients on similar topics.

In preparation for role playing the teacher should

1. Explain the behavioral objective.
2. Explain the process involved in role playing and the procedure.
3. Identify the characters in the situation.
4. Identify the observers.
5. Describe the role of the characters in the role play.
6. Describe the role of the observers.
7. Explain that the characters never rehearse for role playing. The reaction is spontaneous.
8. Explain that at any point during the dramatization the participants may hold a short conference to clarify the problem under study.
9. Explain that the discussion that follows the presentation of the solutions to the problems will be on the learning outcomes that helped students achieve the behavioral objective of the lesson.
10. Indicate that the tape recording that will be made will be available for review by the students.

Listening, Speaking, Reading, and Writing

Abilities in listening, speaking, reading, and writing are generally assumed on the college level of education. However, many adults function at a comparatively low level in these abilities. These four learning activities are dominantly in the cognitive domain. Listening and speaking are complex learned communication behaviors and usually teachers think there is no need to direct teaching of these skills on a post-high-school level of education. However, listening is more than hearing, it involves a receptive attitude. The expression "He will not listen to me" is rather common. The listener needs to concentrate actively to understand what is being said. One must remember and apply what one has heard. If one does not, the cost of not listening may be high. We should listen for ideas and concentrate on this purpose. If so, active listening will give self-satisfaction and satisfaction to the person who is speaking, be it a patient, a teacher, a fellow student, or anyone else. By doing this you give assurance to the speaker.

There are many ways of improving listening and speaking abilities. Among them are

1. After listening to a discussion on any problem of current interest to him, the student is asked for a list of the questions raised and asked for any questions he would like to have brought up if he had been a participant.
2. After the speaker has finished, the student is asked to write down the main points presented in the lecture. Students form small groups and compare their statements. They will begin to sharpen their listening techniques. Writing helps to focus the listener's attention.
3. Students recognize that the obstacle is within themselves that keeps them from listening. They are asked to analyze the situation, find the causes, and remove them. The following suggestions are useful:
   a. Avoid distractions, cooperate with the teacher and other students.
   b. Let your version wait, look at the speaker, concentrate on what he is saying.
   c. Do one thing at a time, take time to listen, and be sincere in your listening.

Improvement in reading skills and vocabulary building may be achieved by the use of special equipment and materials such as a controlled reader that projects materials for adults at a controlled rate. Learners make fewer eye fixations and fewer regressions. This increases the span of recognition. Vocabulary building in nursing and health education may be improved by using the special lists of vocabulary for each subject and the accompanying taped versions.

Learning activities in nursing involve students in written communications. The value of the written record in health care is of major importance. Other means of communication are used but the permanence of the written record makes accuracy and clarity essential.

Writing activities in nursing and health include taking notes in lectures, term papers, projects, descriptions of patients' conditions on charts, day patient reports, conference reports, notes on patient teaching, and self-evaluation notes.

Students may participate in in-service courses in writing on points of special importance in nursing. In writing these records, organization, accurate descriptions, and legibility are stressed. The accurate performance of certain tasks in nursing is essential, but the accurate written description of them and their results is also essential.

The writer of reports in nursing should

1. Avoid abbreviations.
2. Practice building good vocabulary.
3. Practice conciseness.
4. Use formal report forms.
5. Make the message clear.
6. Make the message accomplish the purpose.
7. Plan to evaluate her own written record to see if it meets the standards required in the behavioral objective.

The Workshop

In a workshop participants can work together in small groups on problems that are common to the members of a large group. The purpose of the small groups is to present an opportunity to all the members of the large group to participate and to contribute.

The workshop provides an opportunity for individuals in a large group to learn by doing. The participant studies a problem of his own choice, and the small group organization requires active participation of the individuals. Responsibility has been shifted from teacher to the learner. The learner becomes aware that it is his responsibility to contribute to the solution of the problem.

Workshops are often sponsored by organizations, or by the School of Nursing for study of the curriculum. Workshops are also used to study methods of teaching nursing and health. Participation in this type of experience is valuable in achieving behavioral objectives of a social or democratic nature. The participants have an opportunity to plan together, and to work with other people.

The size of the membership varies according to the purpose of the workshop. The workshop can extend from a day to a week or longer. Workshops sometimes have consultants or resource people to guide and assist them.

The basic unit of the workshop is the small discussion group, with approximately six to ten participants. Workshops may have four or more such units. Each basic unit appoints a chairperson, a secretary, and an observer. At the close of the session each day and at the completion of the workshop, the group summarizes the results of the discussion and the secretary presents the report to the entire membership.

The purpose of the workshop as a learning activity is to teach people to become self-reliant, independent problem solvers. Attendance at, and participation in, a workshop offers learning activities that would help achieve many behavioral objectives. The activities are rich in affective and cognitive learnings. It is an excellent experience for a student to attend a workshop that is successful. The learning outcomes including those gained from planning and working together toward a specific goal are invaluable.

The Panel

The panel consists of a small group of well-qualified persons engaged in conversation in front of a large audience of students. The participants represent different points of view on the same subject but they do not make speeches. A panel is informal and, to a degree, a spontaneous round-table discussion. It is usually selected for a controversial issue. As the members of the panel and the audience interact, the audience sees the relationship of the different points of view.

The moderator, chairperson, or teacher opens the meeting or class period and introduces the panel members. The moderator then gives an overview of the topic to be presented and states the procedures to be followed and the expected outcomes. The moderator tries not to become a contributor, nor to support points of view of the participants. The moderator or teacher guides and keeps the discussion on the topic, and discourages long speeches. Summaries are made by the moderator or teacher at intervals and at the completion of the panel. Questions are encouraged from the members of the audience and they are directed to individual members of the panel.

Materials for presentation should be planned and organized

before the class meeting, otherwise there may be repetition of content. The learning materials should be planned to help achieve the behavioral objectives selected by the students and teacher.

The panel is an expository mode of teaching and provides information and knowledge in the cognitive domain. Knowledge is on the lower level of cognitive learning. The panel is useful when it is necessary to get across to the learners certain specific information required in a curriculum. Student involvement may be increased by the use of questions sequenced from the less complex to the more complex, such as from recall of information, to its analysis, synthesis, and evaluation.

The Symposium

In a symposium, from two to five speakers each present their viewpoint on the same subject in a short prepared talk. The speakers are selected to represent different viewpoints on the same broad issue or topic.

The symposium requires a skillful teacher or moderator. As in the panel,.the teacher introduces the members of the symposium to the student audience and the topic each member will present. Equal time should be allotted to each member, usually ten minutes. The teacher makes the transitional statements between speeches. The teacher summarizes at the completion of the presentations. She opens the discussion to the student audience and directs the questions to the members of the symposium. Like the panel, the symposium is an expository mode or a telling strategy and provides explanations on a topic or issue essential to the learners' objectives in the cognitive domain.

The Seminar

As a learning activity the seminar provides an opportunity for participation in an organized class that utilizes a scientific approach to the analysis of a problem chosen for discussion. The problem may have originated in a research paper or thesis paper. The major purpose of the inquiry is for the learner to develop intellectual skills related to the reflective process. Both inductive and deductive sequencing of information is used.

In conducting a seminar the environment contributes to the purpose. A motivating learning situation, not too highly organized or too relaxed, is essential. The teacher usually guides the seminar; however, a student may carry out the function under the teacher's guidance.

Student participation in guiding the seminar would involve

1. Defining the problem to be discussed.
2. Relating the problem of discussion to the students' behavioral objectives.
3. Directing and focusing the discussion on the problem.
4. Clarifying expressed ideas.
5. Keeping the discussion at a high level.
6. Planning questions that relate to the problem.
7. Guarding against monopoly of discussion by any member of the seminar.
8. Planning a summary at intervals and relating it to the behavioral objectives.
9. Planning for student self-evaluation of progress toward behavioral objectives.

Participation in seminars helps students become more articulate and develop a more critical point of view and a more organized scientific approach toward issues. This approach extends to their personal and professional activities.

Participation in a seminar requires the utilization of many resources to obtain the data required for the discussion, including textbooks, filmstrips, review of studies, and other resource materials. Students are not given the information but must find it for themselves, and they guide their own inquiry. They may collect data, analyze, synthesize, and evaluate it. Active participation in a seminar should help students attain behavioral objectives in cognitive and affective domains and help develop intellectual skills.

Questions

Asking questions is one of the oldest and most commonly used techniques in teaching. A question is a verbal statement that seeks a response from the learner. A question arouses curiosity and mental activity. It stimulates and directs thinking. It is always available to the teacher. It is estimated that teachers spend from 70 to 80 per cent of their time asking questions. They are used for giving directions, to initiate instruction, to manage classroom activities, and many other purposes. The teacher usually intends the question to stimulate thinking; however, this outcome is not always achieved. It is recognized that most questions require students to recall facts, a few require them to think, and the remaining questions are procedural.

Bloom's *Taxonomy of Educational Objectives* has been used to develop guidelines for formulating questions (as well as instructional objectives), based on the six categories of cognitive learning — knowledge, comprehension, application, analysis, synthesis, and evaluation. The teacher can improve the quality of thinking in the classroom by carefully planning questions at all levels of Bloom's taxonomy.

Using Bloom's strategy the teacher may decide to ask questions on the knowledge level, for example, "When was diabetes mellitus discovered?" However, he may wish to increase the level of thinking by asking a question on the application level, such as "Given the present situation, how would you improve the nursing care of Mr. Smith, Unit VI, whose diagnosis is diabetes mellitus?" He may wish to ask a question on the evaluation level, such as "How have Mr. Smith's symptoms changed since his medications have been changed?" This pacing of questions is extremely important where the teaching strategy involves the mastery of a sequence of cognitive skills. Ample time should be spent on each step so that premature lifting of thought to the next level will be guarded against. If premature lifting of thought occurs, fewer and fewer students will participate as discussion continues. The discussion will break down and instead of ending on a high level, it will no doubt return to the lowest level, which is the giving of information.

A teacher may increase a student's awareness by probing to get a rationale for the initial answer by asking another question, such as "What do you mean?" The teacher may refocus the student's response by asking "How does this relate to so and so?" Prompting may also be used if a student cannot answer a question, such as "Why is there a 'no smoking' sign on the unit of Mrs. Smith, who is receiving oxygen?" If the student cannot answer the question, the teacher may ask "Why is there not a 'no smoking' sign on patients' units where oxygen is not being administered?"

Good questions provide for different levels of thinking. Clarity of thought is essential. The question should be stated so that there is no doubt about its purpose. The words should relate meaningfully to the learning activity or experience of the student or learner. Good questions are used as guidelines for the response and therefore should be carefully stated. Questions are used to determine achievement toward behavioral objectives and the learner depends greatly on the quality of the question. If used effectively, questions contribute to the development of desirable attitudes, sustain interest in the subject, and give quality and purpose to the evaluation in the attainment of behavioral objectives. The effectiveness of the use of questions is almost entirely dependent on the teacher's skill in formulating and utilizing them. If skill in using questions is developed, it has great potential in the management of learning as well as the development of student critical thinking.

PLANS FOR TEACHING

The written plan provides information on behavioral objectives and learning activities. It can be used for immediate explanation to the students for their acceptance. A written plan for teaching also serves as a record that can be reviewed and later revised.

The written plan is a product of specific thinking in advance of the teaching period. Time allotment should be distributed in proportion to importance to cognitive, affective, and psychomotor learning. It should also be distributed among different methods of presentation. Students get tired of the same thing; for instance, it may be unwise to devote an entire class period to discussion. Unless it is an extremely provocative topic, interest may be lost before the class period is finished.

Writing a lesson plan affords an opportunity for the teacher to consider relationships of the immediate subject content to the purpose and the general objectives of the curriculum. The plan should present alternate routes or learning experiences, leading to the achievement of the student's behavioral objectives. The teacher must keep in mind that the behavioral objectives must be accepted by the students as their objectives and they must also decide which route should lead most effectively to their objectives.

Planned presentation makes it possible for the teacher to concentrate on what she will do next and give more time and attention to observation, guidance, and student feedback, both verbal and nonverbal. The written plan should not be in great detail and it should be flexible and adjustable to meet the developments in the lesson.

The written plan may be divided into five parts:

1. The objectives, behaviorally stated.
2. Subject content, sufficient in scope, balance, and sequence.
3. Learning activities to provide for student involvement and feedback.
4. A summary, to yield data for generalizations and predictions.
5. An assignment, to provide application and continuity.

A lesson plan can have one or more specific objectives and a series of lessons can contribute to only one objective. For example, the objective "Given a situation in a medical unit in Hospital X, the learner should be able to administer proper medication to a patient with hypertensive heart disease. Criterion determined by the written order on the order sheet and the Hospital Medication Manual," has four or more subordinate objectives that contribute to the main behavioral objective. Each of these four subordinate objectives could be an objective for a lesson plan that would contribute to the competency "Administration of proper medication to a patient with hypertensive heart disease." More than one of these behavioral objectives could be used for one lesson plan.

The teacher should divide the time available among the lessons when more than one lesson contributes to an objective. When more than one teacher shares the presentation, the teacher needs to be aware of the time limits in planning and the over-all presentation so that lessons may be completed without "borrowing" time from the next lesson in the sequence. When a series of lessons contribute to an objective, a lesson should be planned for each subordinate objective. Each lesson should be presented as a complete lesson. It should begin with the presentation of the behavioral objective or objectives, followed by the alternate routes or approaches to the achievement of each objective. It should be completed by a summary or grouping of the data to make it possible for the students to reach their highest level of learning and evaluate their own achievement. Some students may reach the level of evaluation in the cognitive domain and others may not exceed the application level, but students should become accustomed to evaluating their own levels of achievement and the correct terminology that applies to these levels. If this pattern is followed, the domain-referenced grading (see Chapter 10) will be more meaningful to the student.

Lesson Plan Outline

Behavioral Objective: Statement (including competency)

Teacher Activities

1. State the competency.

2. Allocate the content among the three domains of learning: cognitive, affective, and psychomotor.

3. List acceptable levels of learning in the three domains: cognitive — application through evaluation; affective — internalizing, consistently exhibiting; psychomotor — application through integration, with conscious involvement.

   Microlesson: make plan for 5 - 10 minute presentation.

4. Review factors that influence learning.

5. Plan leading questions, such as those beginning with "describe," "enumerate," and "differentiate."

6. Plan assignment, learning outcomes, continuity.

7. Record briefly — feedback.

8. Record names of students who may need additional explanations.

Learning Activities

Plan for student involvement in:

Discussion

Small group activity.

Presentation of summary to group.

Categorization of information.

Development of concepts.

Practice in cognitive, affective, and psychomotor skills.

Analyzing, synthesizing, and evaluating information.

List resources, materials, reading, and teaching aids that are to be used for this lesson.

Sample Lesson Plan

Behavioral Objective: After an assignment in a surgical unit in Hospital X, the student should be able to compile information for the preparation of reports on conditions of patients. Criteria determined by the instructor.

Teacher Activities	*Learning Activities*
1. Competency: "Compile information for the preparation of reports on the condition of patients."	Plan student involvement in:
	How to recognize relevant information, etc.
2. Allocate subject content into the three domains: cognitive, affective, psychomotor.	How to collect data.
	How to organize, evaluate, categorize, and summarize it.
Information:	
relevant irrelevant confidential etc.	Evaluation conference with instructor.
Categorize for written report.	Evaluation of contribution to the replies of leading questions.
3. State acceptable levels of achievement.	Planning learning outcomes for the next meeting.
Microlesson: subordinate relevant objective — "collect and organize data on the conditions of patients in Unit 6."	
4. Review factors that influence learning.	
5. Plan leading questions.	
6. Plan assignment and learning outcomes and continuity.	
7. Record feedback.	
8. Record names of students who may need additional explanations.	

Microlesson

A microlesson is a segment of a regular lesson. It may be a five- or ten-minute portion of a fifty-minute lesson. The objective of the microlesson is a subordinate objective to the objective of the regular lesson. It has all the parts of a regular lesson. It could be the development of a skill such as communication with a patient, or the administration of an injection to a patient. Microlessons build upon a base of knowledge and utilize principles or factors that influence learning as a part of the regular lesson. During the microlesson a videotape recording may be made. At the end of the lesson the student leaves the teaching situation and has a discussion with the supervisor. After the discussion she repeats the lesson with another patient, or members of the patients' family, or a small group of students.

Microlessons are planned as a part of the course in the curriculum. They focus on teaching skills, the mastery of certain curriculum content, or demonstrations of teaching methods. The particular skill is decided on before the teaching period and genuine, not contrived, subject content is utilized.

Microlessons are used in universities in the preparation of teachers in all fields, including medical education in teaching students to work with patients. Microteaching has special significance for nursing education; however, it is important for it to become a specifically organized part of lessons. It should be planned as part of units and lessons throughout the curriculum.

Planned microteaching programs include:

1. Subordinate behavioral objectives for each lesson, including competencies and subordinate competencies.
2. A lesson plan for each microlesson.
3. A unit outline that includes the microlessons, showing levels of progression or sequencing from each semester through the achievement of the behavioral objectives.

Microlessons offer excellent opportunities for students to improve their teaching skills in clinical and community nursing. When videotape recordings are made, students may review them, consider the feedback, analyze it for mistakes, and use the findings for self-evaluation purposes. Microteaching helps to reinforce the students' interest in success and achievement. Microteaching offers opportunities for research and should provide valuable information on teaching consumers of health education and interactions between students, students and teachers, students and patients, and consumers of health care, which could be translated into practice.

Microlesson Plan Outline: 5 — 10 minutes.

Subordinate Behavioral Objective: Statement

Teacher Activities	*Learning Activities*
1. State *subordinate* competency (as stated in the above subordinate objective).	Plan for student involvement: In demonstration of skills: cognitive, affective, or psychomotor.
2. Allocate content among the three domains of learning: cognitive, affective, and psychomotor.	In discussion with patient, students, or other learners.
3. List acceptable levels of achievement.	In analyzing situations and evaluating information.
4. Review factors that influence learning.	In self-evaluation.
5. Plan leading questions such as those beginning with "describe," "explain," and "compare."	In repeat microlesson to develop consistency in performance.
6. Plan continuity of contact with individual or group, and anticipated learning outcomes.	A conference with the teacher follows the microlesson immediately.
7. Students' suggestions for improvement in planning experience (feedback).	

Sample Microlesson Plan: 5 to 10 minutes.

Subordinate Behavioral Objective: After an assignment in Medical-Surgical Nursing, Unit 6, Hospital X, the student should be able to "collect, and organize data on the conditions of patients in Unit 6 in ten minutes."

Criterion: Evaluation conference with instructor.

Teacher Activity	*Learning Activities*
1. Competency — subordinate: "collect data on the conditions of patients in Unit 6."	Plan student involvement in: How to recognize relevant information, etc.
2. Allocate content among the three domains of learning: cognitive, affective, and psychomotor.	How to collect data. How to organize, evaluate, and categorize it, make a decision or diagnosis.
3. List acceptable levels of achievement.	Demonstrate collection, organizing, etc., of data, and recording information from patient's chart.
4. Review factors that influence learning.	
5. Plan leading questions such as those beginning with "describe" and "identify."	Consider factors that influence learning.
6. Plan continuity of contact with individual and group, and learning outcomes.	Examine strategy for positive and negative results.
7. Record feedback.	Refer to return visit or return to group.
8. Result of evaluation conference, repeat performance.	Check feedback from group or patient.

SUMMARY

Tradition reinforces the idea that teachers teach a class rather than individual learners. However, an audience of one thousand still consists of one thousand individuals. It is when a teacher begins to look at individual learners that the differences among them become apparent.

In teaching the challenge is to make effective contact with the individual learner. There is no set formula. Some learners profit more from a visual approach, others from a verbal approach, and other learners profit more from physical activities. Most students will learn from a combination of all the approaches.

Individualized instruction involves adapting procedures to fit each student's needs and to increase his learning possibilities. It may range from minor adaptations in group instruction to provision of independent learning experiences. It may be a variation in objectives to be achieved, learning activities, or criteria for evaluation. The teacher attempts to work with each individual even when one is part of a group. These adaptations and practices represent efforts to allow for individual differences of learners and to help the learners achieve their behavioral objectives more effectively.

In planning teaching-learning strategy, the achievement of the behavioral objective is the measure of success. Learning activities are selected for this achievement. Learning activities are educational exercises that are related to the achievement of the behavorial objective and its competency. They may include observing a demonstration, listening to a lecture, participating in role playing, demonstrating a hypodermic injection of a medication, or listening to a symposium. All learning activities must be justified in terms of their contribution toward the behavioral objectives.

The verb in the competency is the key to the level of learning to be attained by the learner, and the activities that will produce that level should be selected. Steps in the selection of learning activities are illustrated in Figure 8.1. The learning activities are selected according to the composition of the competency and to the dominant domain. An effort should be made to prevent an imbalance of learning activities in any one of the three domains, cognitive, affective, and psychomotor. The purpose of the checklist, Figure 8.2, is to assist in the selection of learning activities and by so doing, to create an awareness of imbalances.

Figure 8.3 shows how one behavioral objective may have a number of competencies, how each competency will have learning activities to be selected according to their dominant domain and level of learning. Descriptions of several learning activities including lecture, demonstration, seminar, and workshop, are provided as suggested means for achievement of behavioral objectives.

The written plan for teaching serves as a record that later can be reviewed. Writing a lesson plan provides an opportunity for the teacher to consider relationships of the immediate subject content to the purpose and objectives of the curriculum and of the lesson. Written plans should be brief but flexible and provide alternate routes that lead to the student's objectives.

Suggested guides for plans to be used for regular and microlessons are included. Microlessons are planned as a part of the regular lesson. The organization of microlessons as part of the units of instruction should be continued over four or five semesters so as to give learners an opportunity to develop expertise in teaching and nursing. Microlessons provide excellent opportunities to meet the individual needs of learners and to make direct contact with them.

REFERENCES

1. Bluming, Mildred, et al., *Solving Teaching Problems*. Pacific Palisades, Calif.: Goodyear Publishing Co., 1973

2. Gronlund, Norman E., *Individualizing Classroom Instruction*. New York: Macmillan Publishing Co., Inc., 1974

3. Guinee, Kathleen K., *The Professional Nurse, Orientation, Roles, and Responsibilities*. New York: Macmillan Publishing Co., Inc., 1970.

4. Hogstel, Mildred O., "A System for Personalized Instruction," *Nursing Outlook,* Vol. 24, No. 2 (February 1976) pp. 110–114.

5. Howes, Virgil M., *Informal Teaching in the Open Classroom*. New York: Macmillan Publishing Co., Inc., 1974.

6. Joyce, Bruce, *Models of Teaching*. Englewood Cliffs, N. J.: Prentice-Hall, Inc., 1972.

7. Keller, Fred S., "Good-Bye Teacher," *Journal of Applied Behavior Analysis,* Vol. 1, No. 1 (Spring 1968), pp. 79–89.

8. Kennin, J. S., *Discipline and Group Management: Theory and Skill Training*. New York: Macmillan Publishing Co., Inc., 1970.

9. Lange, Crystal, "Securing Funding — The Media Center," *Nursing Outlook,* Vol. 24, No. 6 (June 1976), pp. 338.

10. Lapp, Diane, et al., *Teaching and Learning: Philosophical, Psychological, Curricular Applications,* New York: Macmillan Publishing Co., Inc., 1975.

11. Lifton, Walter M., *Education for Tomorrow, The Role of Media*. New York: John Wiley and Sons, Inc., 1970.

12. Lowenfeld, Viktor, and W. Lambert Brittain, *Creative and Mental Growth,* 6th ed. New York: Macmillan Publishing Co., Inc., 1975.

13. McLuhan, Marshall, *Hot and Cold,* New York: Signet Books, 1969.

14. _____. *Understanding Media,* New York: Signet Books, 1969.

15. Meehan, M. L., "What About Team Teaching?" *Educational Leadership,* Vol. 30, No. 5 (May 1973), pp. 717–720.

16. Paduano, Mary Ann, "Evaluation in the Nursing Laboratory: An Honest Appraisal," *Nursing Outlook,* Vol. 24, No. 11 (February 1976), pp. 702–704.

17. Reilly, Dorothy E., *Behavioral Objectives in Nursing Evaluation of Learner Attainment,* New York: Appleton-Century-Crofts, Division of Prentice-Hall, Inc., 1975.

18. Silberman, Charles, *Crisis in the Classroom.* New York: Random House, Inc., 1970.

19. Simon, Sidney B., et al., *Values Clarification: A Handbook of Practical Strategies for Teachers and Students.* New York: Hart Publishing Co., 1972.

20. Tanner, Daniel, *Using Behavioral Objectives in the Classroom.* New York: Macmillan Publishing Co., Inc., 1972.

21. Travers, Robert M. W., *Essentials of Learning.* Macmillan Publishing Co., Inc., 1967.

22. Wilbur, Muriel Bliss, *Educational Tools for Health Personnel.* New York: Macmillan Publishing Co., Inc., 1968.

Chapter Behavioral Objectives

Using information from Chapter 9 as criteria, the learner should be able to:
1. Describe correctly how to select teaching-learning aids and resources for a given behavioral objective, such as "Given a clinic situation, decide the three most important points a consumer of health should know about tetanus antitoxin. Criteria as stated in the Clinical Manual."
2. Differentiate accurately between the advantages of the use of the overhead projector and the chalkboard as teaching-learning aids.
3. Determine two learning aids you would like to use in the teaching-learning strategy for the behavioral objective stated in No. 1. State reasons for the selection.

At the completion of Chapter 9, given the following behavioral objective, "In a clinic situation, the learner should be able to demonstrate ability to communicate effectively with Mr. Brown, in three statements, why he should receive influenza vaccine. Substantiate each of the three statements. Criteria as stated in the Clinical Manual." Select two learning activities and two teaching-learning aids or resources for each activity that you would use in communicating with Mr. Brown. Defend your decisions in each instance in terms of material presented in Chapter 9.

CHAPTER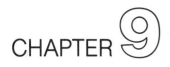

Extension of Learning Activities —
Aids and Resources

AIDS AND RESOURCES

Aids and resources are the learning materials and media selected to extend or supplement learning activities. Various combinations of learning activities, teaching aids, and resources can be used to present a topic. A learning activity, for example, listening to a lecture on drinking water protection, may be extended by showing a motion picture on the functions of a community water purification plant. The motion picture is an aid. If a field trip is planned to the local plant, the trip is the learning activity and the local community water purification plant is the resource. The theme of "clean water for your community" with specific points of interest at the water purification plant may have been presented on the bulletin board, another learning aid in the classroom. Probably the most obvious example of an aid as an extension of the teacher's activity is the microphone. Properly used, the microphone not only enables her to be heard in the back of a large room, but for emphasis, the teacher can vary her voice modulation to a whisper and it can be heard.

SELECTION OF LEARNING AIDS AND RESOURCES

The learning experience should be made as natural as possible or nearly like the situation in which it will be used. Contrived experiences should be used only when natural experiences are not available.

In the selection of learning aids and resources, the teacher should

1. Consider the content of the behavioral objectives to be attained.
2. Consider the learning experience to be extended or supplemented. Is it an accurate, natural, not forced, extension?
3. Consider the factors that influence learning, such as association.
4. Consider the possibility of imbalance of cognitive, affective, and psychomotor learning.
5. Consider opportunities for feedback.
6. Consider alternate experiences to meet individual differences of students.

VISUAL AIDS

The Bulletin Board

As a teaching aid, the bulletin board is used to display information related to the achievement of behavioral objectives of students and teachers. These objectives may be of a lesson, a course, or a unit of instruction. One bulletin board may have information on the daily lessons, and another bulletin board may have a display related to the objectives of a particular unit of instruction.

If the behavioral objective should read "The learner, at the completion of Lesson VI, should be able to correctly evaluate the health education needs in a certain segment of a particular community. Criteria determined by the information in textbook, article, lecture, and information or theme presented on the bulletin boards." The theme on the bulletin board could include pictures of the particular community showing poor housing and flooded streets after a recent rainstorm. The student links the conditions in the community with poor housing and poor sanitation. The student associates the needs of the people in the community with their need for health education and relates these activities to their behavioral objectives.

A bulletin board may be made of cork, beaverboard, or other materials that make it easy to attach items for display. It should be properly lighted and the display should attract the interest of the passer-by. Color scheme can be combined with the information.

Placed on eye level, the printing or writing should be large enough to be easily seen.

Responsibility for the display may be accepted by individuals or small groups of students. Producing the theme requires creativity, interest, and industry. The focus must be kept on the behavioral objectives and their achievement. The learning materials on the bulletin board must be integrated into the whole learning plan.

The Magnetic Board

Magnetic boards have a backing of metal. When small magnets are adhered to the back of the display materials, they will hold to the board. These boards are light in weight and can be carried from place to place and changed to meet the needs of the teacher. A magnetic board is also helpful in teaching patients who are confined to bed. It is a very useful aid for microlessons.

The Felt Board and the Flannel Board

The felt or flannel board may be used in combination with the bulletin board or a chalkboard. Flannel or felt boards are made by covering a heavy cardboard with the selected material. Pictures, letters of the alphabet, or other display materials with felt, flannel, or sandpaper on the back can be stuck to this board. Display materials such as pictures of resuscitation methods, or equipment, or diagrams showing statistics are easily mounted on pieces of sandpaper that will adhere to the flannel or felt board. Visual aids such as the exhibit on the magnetic board or the flannel board must be selected to supplement the learning activities that will contribute to the cognitive, affective, and psychomotor aspects of the behavioral objectives of the lesson.

The Chalkboard

The chalkboard is an accepted part of the classroom and it is an important aid in teaching. It provides a means to present ideas or information to meet the teacher and student needs that may arise during the lesson. The need may be an explanation of a new medical term. The teacher may turn, write the word on the board, pronounce it, and then give an explanation of it. Another use may be in a reply to a question from a student. The teacher may wish to substantiate her answer by using statistics and a diagram. Spontaneously she can turn to the chalkboard because it is available, and present the material. It must be kept in mind that the information must be related to the student's needs and achievement of their objectives.

The general appearance of the chalkboard should not be crowded. Information should be organized and framed under headings such as behavioral objectives, competencies, or sub-competencies. If items are not organized on the chalkboard, learners may copy incomplete information in their notebooks. Once information on a chalkboard becomes unnecessary, it should be erased. Otherwise it becomes a visual distraction.

The teacher should write legibly on the chalkboard and then stand out of the students' line of vision so that they may see it. She also has to give them sufficient time to copy the material in their notebooks before she erases it.

The Overhead Projector

In recent years, the overhead projector has developed into a popular and versatile teaching tool. It is one of the most flexible methods for visual communication in the classroom. Use of the overhead projector allows the presenter or teacher to remain in the normal speaking position in the front of the room and yet maintain control over the visual material. The teacher can select her own pace, extemporize as she wishes, and answer questions or comment before or after the projection.

The overhead projector is easy to operate. There are only four controls — on, off, one to lower or raise the image, and a knob to focus the picture. The projector consists basically of a lighted horizontal stage upon which transparencies are placed and a specifically designed lens that projects the material on a screen. A screen on the wall, on a tripod, or a chalkboard may be used. The projector light source is sufficient to provide good screen illumination without having to darken the room. The proper placement of the overhead projector is in the front of the room with the projector low and the screen high. The angle of the projection should allow the students or other learners to see over the head of the presenter and over the projector. Transparencies generally consist of a sheet of clear acetate approximately 8-½ × 11 inches. Commercially prepared transparencies come in sets of ten to twenty. These should be carefully reviewed to determine the appropriateness to the course or lesson. Overlays may be used to build ideas from simple to complex. This may be accomplished by using a basic visual and superimposing several sheets of film to build up a number of components into a composite image. For instance, it is possible to project an outline of a lung, and then superimpose the circulation of the organ.

The overhead projector can be used instead of a chalkboard. The same words and diagrams that the teacher would ordinarily write on the chalkboard are written on a blank acetate sheet with a marking pencil. This approach is useful when the group being addressed is large or spread out in a large room such as an auditorium, since the projection becomes an "enlarged chalkboard," easy for all to see.

In teaching, the advantages of overhead projection are many. When a particular behavioral objective calls for the development of cognitive behavior in systematic instruction, projectuals combined with lecture-discussion, when used skillfully, should help students and teachers achieve this goal.

Microprojector

The teacher of nursing frequently uses microscopic slides as subject content in lectures. To present these slides, projection equipment that incorporates a microscope can make it possible for large numbers of students to directly view the actual microscopic slides as they are projected on a screen. The directions should be carefully read to be certain that heat does not damage the slides.

The Textbook

The textbook is the most commonly used learning aid. It is utilized as a major information source in most courses of instruction. Textbooks should be supplemented by reading materials from other sources, such as journals, and also by lectures. The teacher synthesizes information from several textbooks.

Courses of study and curriculum guides are useful in curriculum development, and textbooks provide the teacher with a presentation of sequenced materials that are organized and focused on a specific goal or purpose. This presentation of sequenced content can be examined by the teacher and the student. It presents a position on the subject resulting from study and conviction that it is usable and effective in helping students and teachers achieve their goals.

Models, Objects, Specimens, and Exhibits

Models, objects, and specimens provide multisensory opportunities for students to see an object, touch it, feel it, and handle it. In this direct learning experience, the student perceives the object as it actually exists.

Models

A model is a representation of something, life-size, enlarged, or miniature. It may be an articulated skeleton or a life-size model of the body showing the different parts. Anatomical models can be taken apart, studied, and then put together again. The parts of models usually correspond in dimension to the average size and shape of the parts of the body. Such models are helpful in the study of anatomy and physiology and nursing.

Equipment

In teaching nursing, there are many pieces of equipment such as the sphygmomanometer, stethescope, otoscope, respirators, and other objects essential in giving nursing care. Students may become familar with them before their learning experiences extend to the clinical nursing situation.

Specimens

Specimens such as a dissected heart are used to show the nature and structure of the organ. Each student should carefully examine the specimen made available in this unique opportunity. In study laboratories, these specimens are usually kept in a preserving fluid.

Exhibits

Objects may be arranged in a display to communicate certain ideas or a theme. It could be the emergency care of a person who was admitted to the Emergency Room in coma. The exhibit would include the newest equipment available for use, as well as an endotracheal tube, equipment for intravenous infusion, drugs for the emergency condition, and a respirator. Exhibits are conducive to learning because there is time to examine the objects and ask questions, so that later the students will know how to adjust and use the equipment, which is the first step in psychomotor learning.

AUDIOVISUAL AIDS

Educational Films

Motion pictures bring sight, sound, and motion together. The conventional 16 mm sound film is one of the most commonly used multisensory teaching aids in nursing and health education. There is a great variety of films on nursing and health education available. Many agencies and foundations produce health films. Some may be obtained free of cost and others at little cost. Indeed, there are so many available that selection becomes a problem.

Motion pictures are so easily available that excessive use is likely to occur. Too often, students may be subjected to a "film week" of instruction without previewing preparation or opportunities for discussion. The same film is sometimes shown to the same groups of students on different occasions. Frequently the students prepare for a film on one topic, such as "The First Aid for a Choking Patient," and arrive in the classroom on schedule to find that the film did not come and a substitute film, "The Care of the Newborn," is being shown. Films are also shown to replace scheduled lessons when a teacher may be required to attend a meeting.

A film should be selected only if its content contributes to the achievement of behavioral objectives. Technical perfection alone does not accomplish this goal. The instructor or teacher of nursing is the one who decides on the value of the film and she must first be very clear about the kind of learning required in the objective.

When properly chosen, motion pictures are excellent teaching aids to supplement cognitive, affective, and psychomotor learning activities. One area where motion pictures are particularly helpful in aiding cognitive learning experiences is that of time-lapse and high-speed photography. By use of these simple photographic devices, a natural phenomenon that may have taken hours or days can be visually presented in minutes, and conversely, an episode that occurs in seconds can be lengthened to minutes for ease of observation. Time lapse is often used to show such processes as cell division, motion of phagocytes, and the development or healing of a lesion. A familiar example of high-speed photography is the visual recording of a car crashing into a barrier and the effectiveness of seat belts and other safety devices.

Educational films may also be used to develop affective learning. The sound film is an excellent medium when used to convey the attitudes of people — physicians, nurses, patients, and others. These attitudes may be expressed by sound or facial expressions, the latter made more intense by visual close-ups. The emotional content of educational films should be well balanced with accurate information and interpreted properly in relation to the behavioral objectives.

Films can be used to direct students in the acquisition of psychomotor skills. For example, a short film showing a cross section of tissues can be used in teaching the administration of medication by hypodermic or by intramuscular injection. The film would show the needle as it passes through the different layers of tissue. In this instance, after the film is used to introduce the topic, provision must be made for further instruction, feedback, practice, and evaluation.

The selection of the film must include consideration of the level of learning involved, which is determined by the verb in the competency, such as analysis, synthesis, evaluation, or other levels in cognitive, affective, and psychomotor domains. In nursing, the behavioral objectives could involve the evaluation of the type of health education that should be used for a particular community portrayed in the accompanying motion picture. The content should represent that indicated in the competency and subcompetencies of the behavioral objectives. Information on the content is obtained from the film description, and other sources; however, the final selection is not made until the film is previewed. When the teacher previews a film, she should note relevant points that will form the basis of questions or discussion. It is useful to keep a film card file for future reference, which incorporates these notes as well as comments on the impact on the students when shown.

The following are some suggestions that simplify the presentation of a film and influence learning outcomes:

1. The film should be presented at the appropriate time within the lesson. It must be incorporated into the existing teaching pattern.
2. The behavioral objectives of the lesson should be reviewed. The learners will then know what they are supposed to be looking

for and the relevant points in the film. This guide can be verbal or printed.

3. The students should not plan to take notes. If they do, they cannot concentrate on the content of the film.

4. The teacher should provide an opportunity and time for feedback.

5. The teacher should summarize the high points relevant to the objectives.

6. The students should summarize the presentation of the lesson including the content presented in the film, incorporating it into the entire lesson and plan for evaluation.

7. The teacher should cooperate with the Visual-Aid Department by ordering teaching aids in advance and returning them immediately following the presentation in the classroom, so that the equipment will be available for other teachers.

Lantern Slides

Lantern slides have been used over a period of time in classrooms. Many excellent automatic remote control projectors are available for these pictures. They are relatively small and easy to carry from room to room and also easy to store. Most schools of nursing are situated in colleges or universities and share the projection equipment and slides with other departments, through a central facility. The teacher should preview the pictures before they are selected as a teaching aid to the learning activity, that is, a lecture, discussion, panel, or other activity that can be extended by related pictures. The content of the slides must be integrated into the lecture materials that are selected to help students achieve their objectives.

Lantern slides are 3-½ × 4 inches and can be made by students and the teacher. These glass slides may be purchased from a commercial firm. Statistics or other information may be typed on a special film and placed on the slide. Graphs, or other information may be placed on a special tape that is attached to the slide. Information may also be written directly on the slide. There is a large area of the slide that the light passes through and, as a result, the room is bright enough for students to take notes.

Filmstrips

Filmstrips have pictures placed in sequence on a roll of 35 mm film instead of separate slides. Each picture is called a "frame." The filmstrip is valuable when observation and study of a frame is necessary. The filmstrip is particularly suitable for individual study. It is very useful in a step-by-step procedure in nursing. A recorded commentary may parallel the filmstrip, and this too can be controlled while observing a particular frame.

Slides

Slides are easy to obtain because of the simplicity of the modern 35 mm camera. When the picture is developed, it is mounted as a slide and comes ready for use. Series of slides on special topics may be purchased, but the teacher can also collect her own slides. Automatic control projectors are used for presentation. The teacher comments on each slide as it is projected. A few slides may be selected to supplement discussion or other activity. The content of slides is easy to integrate into the entire lesson.

Audio Devices

There are many occasions when the use of audio resources could help communicate the information to be presented in nursing and health education. Audio devices may be used in isolation or in conjunction with visual aids. The tape recorder may be used in recording group conferences or lectures. It may also be used in group presentations and can be incorporated into a lesson.

The tape recorder may be used to record patient interviews, reports, and class discussions. It is a very versatile device because it can be played back to the class or it may be used for self-evaluation. In this instance, criteria must be established against which the student may judge her performance. It is an excellent means of motivation for students and teachers to improve their discussion and speaking skills. Teachers as well as students should make use of the tape recorder for this purpose.

Tape recordings of lectures are frequently used by students for individual projects. When they have been unable to attend a lecture, they can replay a tape made by the instructor or another student.

Just as vision may be extended by films, so may hearing be extended by recording on tape or disc. Auditory sensations play an important part in educational programs in nursing and health education. There are sounds every nurse should recognize. The American Heart Association, as well as several other organizations,

have released a series of high fidelity recordings of normal and abnormal heart sounds as aids to teaching auscultation of the heart.
Other recordings that feature different experts discussing specific
topics are helpful to students of nursing in achievement of their
behavioral objectives and they may become an essential aid to the
lesson. In many areas of the United States, an extensive series of
educational tape recordings on cancer are available by toll-free
phone call.

Videotape cassettes covering a wide range of topics are now
available. These can be used with projection equipment in the same
manner as a motion picture. The same cassette presented to the class
can be made available to the student in a library videotape carrel or
room for review at a later time. Videotapes are particularly useful
for viewing by a single student as part of an individualized learning
plan.

Television

Television is a powerful means of audiovisual communication. It
does not replace the teacher; rather it combines all teaching media.
It may bring into the classroom lectures by prominent physicians
and teachers of nursing and health. Television as a teaching aid in
nursing education must be well planned and closely coordinated.

Television has played a role in medical education, particularly
in surgery and special diagnostic techniques. In surgery it offers to
many students the advantage and immediacy that could otherwise be
achieved by only one or two. The view from a raised platform, twenty or more feet away, cannot be compared with that transmitted
from a camera in the overhead light, beamed at the operative site.
This view can be magnified to convenience as well. This same
procedure allows students of nursing to observe operating
procedures.

A closed-circuit television system can be used as a "one way
mirror." A small camera can transmit an interview between a
patient and a professional to be viewed by an entire class. This
allows all the students the opportunity to have contact with the
patient in a real situation and yet the patient does not have to be put
on a stage, so to speak. In this situation, of course, the patient is told
that the students are watching in another room and the patient's permission is required.

Television has been used successfully in in-service courses for personnel working in different buildings or hospitals in a city. In these instances, a single skilled teacher is able to reach many small groups using teaching aids and resources available only at the central location. A teacher or discussion leader should be present at each of the receiving sites to highlight the objectives of the presentation and guide their local application.

Television must adhere to a specific time schedule, and the teacher must conform to that time schedule if she is going to utilize it as a part of the lesson. If a television program is going to be used, it is best to plan it for the first part of the class period, to allow for student-teacher discussion and questions.

In public health education, television is used to bring information to the public in feature programs on such topics as kidney dialysis, detection of cancer, or progress in cardiac surgery. It is also used to change the attitude of people toward venereal and other diseases. The purpose of many short news feature programs on television is to inform the public on positive health practices.

In utilizing television as a teaching aid, the teacher should

1. Review the behavioral objectives of the lesson.
2. Review the content of the program before it is presented, if this is possible.
3. Use only television that will present material you cannot present more effectively by other means.
4. Plan for questions and discussion following the presentation.
5. Consider factors that influence learning, such as perception.
6. Take notes on cognitive and affective learning and plan for immediate practice for psychomotor skills shown.
7. Remember television is a "one-shot" performance and there is no repeat performance.

RESOURCES

Part of the teacher's responsibility is to facilitate the exposure of the student to a wide range of learning experiences, many of which are not and cannot be centered on the classroom. She must look to resources both intramurally and extramurally. Further, she must know and be reasonably familiar with these resources if they are to be properly utilized.

The first "on campus" intramural resource that comes to mind is the library. Aside from general reference texts, the library will most often reflect the needs of the potential users. Thus large sections on medicine or pharmacology would be expected in a library that serves schools of medicine and pharmacy as well as the school of nursing. The proximity of patient care facilities in hospital inpatient services and clinics are also necessary resources.

Often the teacher will be able to take advantage of the facilities of other departments, such as teaching machines in the education laboratories and audiovisual materials and equipment in the Communications Department.

It should be mentioned that one of the advantages of being on a college campus is the availability of an extracurricular program. The teacher should encourage her students to participate in such activities as dramatics, sports, and the university radio station.

Traditionally, the extramural resources most often tapped by schools of nursing are the local health department and the visiting nurse service. In these settings, the student becomes more aware of how the day-to-day priorities of the community affect the delivery of health care.

Other hospitals, aside from the parent hospital, should not be forgotten as resources. Especially now with the emphasis on planning health facilities, hyperbaric oxygen chambers, expensive radiation therapy centers, and burn centers are not being duplicated in every city. Knowing where these special facilities are and making them available to her students is becoming a more important aspect of the teacher's job.

Field visits to industrial plants are used to deal primarily with the employee health and accident prevention program. Now students and teachers are emphasizing protection of the worker's health as well as that of the surrounding community. Many of the larger industrial sites have initiated programs for protection against toxic substances being used. A company physician, occupational hygienist, or safety officer is often available to explain these developments.

SUMMARY

Aids and resources are the learning materials and media selected to extend or supplement learning activities. The learning activity of listening to a lecture on a safer water supply may be extended by a visit to a community location such as a water purification plant. The plant is the resource. A theme, "Clean Water for your Community," with specific points of interest at the purification plant may be presented on the bulletin board, an aid.

Learning aids and resources are selected primarily for their contribution to the achievement of the students' behavioral objectives. Various types of aids and resources may be used to fit the individual needs of learners. Selection of aids and resources includes consideration of a balance of cognitive, affective, and psychomotor learning, provision for feedback, and other factors that influence learning.

Visual aids, such as the bulletin board, magnetic board, and the felt board, are supplementary to the chalkboard and the materials or theme included on these boards should be integrated into the content of the lecture or other learning activity of which it is an extension. The overhead projector, one of the most versatile teaching tools, is a great asset to the lecture as an extension and increases the possibilities for the achievement of behavioral objectives. The textbook, the most commonly used learning aid, should be supplemented by reading materials from other sources such as journals, and also by lectures.

Audiovisual aids including educational films, when properly chosen, are excellent teaching aids to supplement cognitive, affective, and psychomotor learning activities. They involve multiple senses by bringing pictures, sound, and motion together. They are particularly helpful in presenting cognitive learning experiences, such as cell division, by simple photographic devices. Processes that may take hours or days can be presented in minutes, and conversely an episode that occurs in seconds can be lengthened to minutes for ease of observation. Lantern slides, filmstrips, and slides may be used with or without sound recordings. The teacher may wish to give a commentary and integrate the content of these aids into the lecture or discussion.

Sound recordings are extensions of hearing and play an important part in educational programs in nursing and health education. Television also plays a major role. Closed-circuit television has proved very successful in teaching students of nursing and also in-service education programs where one teacher may reach many people in many different locations.

REFERENCES

1. American Nurses Association, *The Professional Nurse and Health Education*. Kansas City, Mo.: A.N.A., 1975, pp. 1–7.

2. American Nurses Association, *Standards, Nursing Practice*. Kansas City, Mo.: A.N.A., 1973.

3. Bevis, E., *Curriculum Building in Nursing — A Process*. St. Louis, Mo.: The C.V. Mosby Company, 1973.

4. Dineen, M. A., "The Open Curriculum: Implications for Further Education," *Nursing Outlook,* Vol. 20, No. 12 (December 1972), p. 770.

5. Gagne, Robert M., *Conditions of Learning*. New York: Holt, Rinehart and Winston, 1965.

6. Gronlund, Norman E., *Individualizing Classroom Instruction*. New York: Macmillan Publishing Co., Inc., 1974.

7. _____, *Stating Behavioral Objectives for Classroom Instruction*. New York: Macmillan Publishing Co., Inc., 1970.

8. Howes, Virgil M., *Informal Teaching in the Open Classroom*. New York: Macmillan Publishing Co., Inc., 1974.

9. Johnson, Lois V., et al., *Classroom Management: Theory and Skill Training*. New York: Macmillan Publishing Co., Inc., 1969.

10. Lifton, Walter M., *Education for Tomorrow, The Role of Media*. New York: John Wiley and Sons, Inc., 1970.

11. Lange, Crystal, "Securing Funding — The Media Center," *Nursing Outlook,* Vol. 24, No. 6 (June 1976), p.351.

12. Litwack, Lawrence, "A System of Evaluation," *Nursing Outlook,* Vol. 24, No. 1 (January 1976), pp.45–58.

13. McLuhan, Marshall, *Hot and Cold,* New York: Signet Books, 1969.

14. _____, *Understanding Media,* New York: Signet Books, 1969.

15. Mager, Robert F., et al., *Analyzing Performance Problems*. Belmont, Calif.: Fearon Publishers, 1970.

16. *Nursing Outlook,* "A System for Personalized Instruction," Vol. 24, No. 2 (February 1976), pp. 110–114.

17. Plowman, Paul D., *Behavioral Objectives*. Chicago, Ill.: Science Research Associates, Inc., 1971.

18. Popham, Estelle L., Adele Frisbee Schrag, and Wanda Blockus, *A Teaching-System for Business Education*. New York: Gregg Division, McGraw-Hill Book Company, 1975.

19. Popham, James W., et al., *Planning Instructional Sequence*. Englewood Cliffs, N.J.: Prentice-Hall, Inc., 1970.

20. Read, Donald A., et al., *Creative Teaching in Health,* 2nd ed. New York: Macmillan Publishing Co., Inc., 1975.

21. Schweer, J. E., *Creative Teaching in Clinical Nursing,* 2nd ed. St. Louis, Mo.: The C. V. Mosby Company, 1972.

22. Skinner, B. F., *The Technology of Teaching.* New York: Appleton-Century-Crofts, 1968.

23. Tanner, Daniel, *Using Behavioral Objectives in the Classroom.* New York: Macmillan Publishing Co., Inc., 1972.

24. Tyler, Ralph W., et al., *Perspectives on Curriculum Evaluation.* Chicago, Ill.: Rand-McNally & Co., 1967.

25. Wilbur, Muriel Bliss, *Educational Tools for Health Personnel.* New York: Macmillan Publishing Co., Inc., 1968.

26. Wright, Kenneth B., et al., *Career Education: What It Is and How to Do It.* Salt Lake City, Utah: Olympus Publishing Co., 1972.

Chapter Behavioral Objectives

At the completion of Chapter 10, the learner should be able to

1. Decide which evaluation device should be used for the following behavioral objectives: "While being observed by a teacher, the student should be able to use data from different sources and make a decision appropriate to the situation. Criterion determined by the teacher." Defend your choice of evaluation device by using material in this chapter.
2. Decide when to use norm-referenced tests in criterion-referenced instruction. Criteria according to information in Chapter 10.
3. Determine the dominant domain of the following behavioral objective: "At the completion of the unit on the administration of medications, the student should be able to explain correctly what causes drugs to form a precipitate. Criteria determined by the instructor."
4. Differentiate between the purpose of formative tests and the purpose of summative tests. Criteria as stated in Chapter 10.
5. Make a checklist for evaluation of an individual's performance incorporating the levels of learning in the affective domain. Criteria as stated in Chapter 10.

CHAPTER 1

Grading the Attainment
of Behavioral Objectives

EVALUATION AND GRADING

Schools require a record of the attainments of students for entrance and the school is expected to produce a record of the student's accomplishments when she leaves or graduates. To provide data for this record, a system of evaluation that measures the learner's achievement toward stated behavioral objectives must be established and maintained.

There are many ways of grading student achievements but generally there must be uniformity as well as flexibility in the grading system of a school of nursing so as to conform to the system used by the college or university of which it is a part.

Evaluation is a basic element in a teaching-learning program in nursing education. The purpose of evaluation is to determine how much the student has achieved and to find out if she possesses the foundation for new knowledge. As we have noted, pretesting is used to determine the student's status at the beginning of the course or unit of instruction. At the completion of the unit of instruction, posttests are given. Chapter objectives may be used for the pretest and also for the posttest. The student's achievement will be the difference between the results of the pretest and the results of the posttest. The pretest itself may be used for the posttest. If the same examination is not used for both the pretest and posttest, the new test must mirror the pretest. Without this information the teacher would be unable to guide the learner in her achievement of increasingly more complex material.

NORM-REFERENCED AND CRITERION-REFERENCED EVALUATION AND GRADING

Either norm-referenced or criterion-referenced evaluation, or a combination of the two, may be used to measure achievement in nursing education. In a norm-referenced system of evaluation, the student's achievement on a test is measured in relation to the achievement of other students who took the test. Criterion-referenced tests measure an individual student's achievement toward a specific standard stated in the behavioral objective. The type of test used must be valid for the objectives and their competencies in nursing. See Chapters 4 and 5. Whichever strategy is used it must be appropriate to the behavioral objective to be attained and the competency that is to be developed.

Norm-referenced evaluation may be used on the minimum essentials level, such as recall of knowledge. In the cognitive domain, this minimum level of attainment would not be considered an acceptable grade for achievement of behavioral objectives in nursing education. Where behavioral objectives, including the statement of competencies, are used as the standard of performance, criterion-referenced tests and domain-referenced grading should be used. The specific criterion stated in the behavioral objective provides an absolute standard against which to compare an individual's achievement.

The objective's major competency determines the dominant domain to be evaluated. With the objective "While being observed by a teacher, the student should be able to decide upon a nursing diagnosis, using data from observations and examinations of the patient. Criteria determined by the teacher," achievement also includes the development of attitudes in the affective domain. In addition, the student will have exhibited psychomotor skill in collecting data, involving the examination of the patient. However, the dominant domain is the category where the grade should be recorded. The findings related to the affective and psychomotor domains should not be lost. They should be recorded on a similar record used for achievements in second and third domains. These and other observations are important to the student and also to the teacher in a system that is individual and sensitive. The student should be shown these evaluations.

CRITERION-REFERENCED TESTS

Gronlund outlines two types of tests that are used for criterion-referenced testing.[1] *Formative* tests may be given at the achievement of subordinate behavioral objectives, for diagnostic purposes, and to provide information to be used to improve methods and materials as the student is progressing toward her objectives. *Summative* tests are given at the end of the course or as a final examination. The emphasis in these tests is on criterion-referenced evaluation. As has been mentioned in Chapter 6, when the student and the teacher decide on the behavioral objectives to be achieved, plans are made for discussions at intervals with each student to discuss her progress toward the behavioral objectives. This makes it possible for a teacher to use the feedback to improve her instruction and to make changes, if necessary.

Criterion-referenced test items should be

1. Written for each behavioral objective.
2. Written for the dominant domain.
3. Checked to see if they are related to the learning outcomes.
4. Checked to see if items are written for each of the different levels of complexity within the dominant domain.
5. Checked to determine if the items test the established criterion of the behavioral objective.

When the results of the test are scored, and percentage or letter grades or symbols affixed, the results should be compared with the required level of the learning outcomes for each behavioral objective, to determine if the behavioral objective has been achieved by the student. The grade may then be recorded on the domain-referenced grading form, Figure 10.1, by indicating "S" on the level of learning required and stated in the behavioral objective.

In observation of individual performance, the teacher will have a checklist of the behavioral objectives and the expected learning outcomes. In addition, she should have a list of the levels of learning in each domain. At the time of the observation, information required for grading should be checked. Grades from the

[1]Gronlund, Norman E. *Preparing Criterion-Referenced Tests for Classroom Instruction* (New York: Macmillan Publishing Co., Inc., 1973), pp. 43–44.

achievement of these objectives should be recorded in the appropriate place. After the teacher has used the list of levels of learning a few times, she will rarely need to refer to it. The experienced teacher will automatically think in terms of levels of learning and dominant domains.

FIGURE 10.1. Suggested Domain-Referenced Grading Form for One Behavioral Objective

		Domains of Learning							
		Cognitive			Affective			Psychomotor	
Levels of learning acceptable for achievement of behavioral objectives:		Application	Analysis and Synthesis	Evaluative	Valuing	Organizing	Internalizing	Acquisition	Application	Integration
Statement of behavioral objective: "While being observed by a teacher, the student should be able to decide upon a nursing diagnosis, using data from different sources. Criteria determined by the teacher."	Approx. Grades 100 A 90 B 80 C									

Signatures:

Teacher

Student

Date

Transfer grade to summary record

DOMAIN-REFERENCED GRADING

Figure 10.1 presents a grading form for the levels of learning that are acceptable for grading in the domain-referenced system, using the cognitive, affective, and psychomotor domains. This form presents a behavioral objective for evaluation in the dominant domain or category of learning: "While being observed by a teacher, the student should be able to decide upon a nursing diagnosis, using data from observations and examination of the patient. Criteria determined by the teacher." The dominant domain of the competency of the behavioral objective is the cognitive domain. If the diagnosis is correctly made, we can assume that the student possesses the appropriate knowledge and can apply it, analyze, synthesize, and evaluate it in the process of making the diagnosis. The achievement of the evaluation level of learning in the cognitive domain presupposes that other levels of learning including knowledge and comprehension were possessed by the student. Acceptable levels of learning are agreed upon by the faculty of the school of nursing.

If a student does not achieve a behavioral objective, the teacher should maintain information on objectives not achieved as well as the levels of learning achieved by these students. This type of record is valuable because of the current emphasis on accountability. It contains the type of information that the teacher needs for a "requested" report on a particular student.

Figure 10.2 shows how more than one domain-referenced grade may be recorded, and Figure 10.3 presents a sample summary record for recording behavioral objectives achieved in a course or unit of instruction. These records show how approximate grades may be used.

SUMMARY

Evaluation is an essential part of an educational program. In criterion-referenced instruction it provides information on the student's progress toward behavioral objectives. This progress can be measured as the difference between the student's achievement on the pretest and the results of the posttest. Evaluation is continuous in criterion-referenced instruction. If a student does not progress as expected, feedback should help to locate the reason for failure. It may be the student's fault, the teacher's fault, or the fault of the

**FIGURE 10.2.   Domain-Referenced Grading Form for More Than One
                Behavioral Objective**

Domains of Learning

Cognitive   Affective   Psychomotor

Levels of learning acceptable for
achievement of behavioral
objectives:

	Application	*Analysis and Synthesis*	*Evaluative*	*Valuing*	*Organizing*	*Internalizing*	*Acquisition*	*Application*	*Integration*

Statements of behavioral   Approx.
Objectives: Grades

1. After completion of the unit   100 A
   of study on classifications
   of drugs, the student should   90 B
   be able to identify correctly
   medications according to   80 C
   their common characteristics.
   Criteria — content from
   textbook for course.

2. At the completion of the unit on the administration of medications the student
   should be able to explain correctly the
   cause-and-effect-relationship between
   medications that combine to form a
   precipitate. Criteria determined by
   instructor.

3. At the completion of Unit 7, the student
   should be able to regularly assemble facts
   and differentiate between relevant and
   irrelevant facts. Criteria determined by
   instructor.

4. After an assignment in a surgical unit,
   the student of nursing should be able to
   compile accurate information for the
   preparation of reports. Criteria determined by instructor.

Transfer Grades to Summary Record

FIGURE 10.3. Sample Summary Record Domain-Referenced Grading

		Domains of Learning								
		Cognitive			*Affective*			*Psychomotor*		
Levels of learning acceptable for achievement of behavioral objectives		*Application*	*Analysis and Synthesis*	*Evaluative*	*Valuing*	*Organizing*	*Internalizing*	*Acquisition*	*Application*	*Integration*
Numbers of behavioral objectives and grades:	Approx. Grades									
	100 A									
	90 B									
	80 C									
	Etc.									

Behavioral Objectives Achieved

Adapted from Estelle Popham, Adele Frisbee Schrag, and Wanda Blockus, *A Teaching — Learning System for Business Education* (New York: McGraw-Hill Book Company, Gregg Division, 1975), p. 157.

teaching-learning strategy. Each possibility should be examined and adjustments made to help the student achieve her behavioral objectives. The effectiveness of the criterion-referenced program may be assessed by noting the number of students who achieve behavioral objectives on the first attempt and the number who need to try to achieve the behavioral objective more than once. Students who achieve higher level behavioral objectives earn higher grades.

In nursing education, criterion-referenced evaluation should be used except when testing for the minimum levels of learning, such as recall of information. Gronlund outlines two types of tests for criterion-referenced programs: (1) formative tests, which may be given at intervals in a course when students achieve certain subordinate objectives — this type of test is also used as feedback and to improve the teaching and testing program — and (2) summative tests, which are given as final examinations.

Criterion-referenced evaluation makes use of written test items, checklists for observation of individual performance, and other measures specifically designed for the evaluation of student progress toward such behavioral objective. Figure 10.1 presents a domain-referenced grading form for recording behavioral objectives achieved at different levels of the cognitive, affective, and psychomotor domains. Figure 10.2 extends the same idea for four objectives that have been achieved, and Figure 10.3 shows a similar form that can be used as a summary record.

Grading is an acceptable requirement in schools of nursing. All systems of grading are less than perfect. The domain-referenced is a relatively objective grading system. If the behavioral objectives are clearly defined and accepted by the teacher and student for achievement on a partnership relationship, it should be possible for the teacher to establish an objective means of measuring student achievement. The domain-referenced grading system does require measurement of achievement of behavioral objectives on levels of cognitive, affective, and psychomotor domains. This specificity should help the teacher in evaluation.

REFERENCES

1. American Cancer Society, Inc., *Cancer Facts and Figures.* New York: American Cancer Society, Inc., 1975, pp. 6–8.

2. American Nurses Association, *The Professional Nurse and Health Education.* Kansas City, Mo.: A.N.A., 1975.

3. American Nurses Association, *Standards, Nursing Practice.* Kansas City, Mo.: A.N.A., 1973.

4. Bell, Terree, "The Means and Ends of Accountability," *Proceedings of the Conference on Educational Accountability.* Princeton, N.J.: Educational Testing Service, 1971.

5. Fivars, G., et al., *Nursing Evaluation: The Problems and the Process.* New York: Macmillan Publishing Co., Inc., 1966.

6. Gronlund, Norman E., *Measurement and Evaluation in Teaching, Instructor's Manual,* 2nd ed. New York: Macmillan Publishing Co., Inc., 1971.

7. _____, *Preparing Criterion-Referenced Tests for Classroom Instruction.* New York: Macmillan Publishing Co., Inc., 1973.

8. _____, *Determining Accountability for Classroom Instruction.* New York: Macmillan Publishing Co., Inc., 1974.

9. _____, *Improving Marking and Reporting in Classroom Instruction.* New York: Macmillan Publishing Co., Inc., 1974.

10. Levinson, Harry, "Appraisal of What Performance?" *Harvard Business Review* Vol. 54, No. 4 (July–August 1976), pp. 30–36.

11. Paduano, Mary Ann, "Evaluation in the Nursing Laboratory: An Honest Appraisal," *Nursing Outlook,* Vol. 22, No. 11 (November 1974), pp. 702–704.

12. Popham, Estelle, Adele Frisbee Schrag, and Wanda Blockus, *A Teaching-Learning System for Business Education.* New York: Gregg Division, McGraw-Hill Book Company, 1975.

13. Popham, James W., *Educational Statistics: Use and Interpretation.* New York: Harper and Row, Publishers, Inc., 1967.

14. Thorndike, Robert L., et al., *Measurement and Evaluation in Psychology and Education,* 3rd ed. New York: John Wiley & Sons, Inc., 1969.

15. Townsend, Edward A., et al., *Using Statistics in Classroom Instruction.* New York: Macmillan Publishing Co., Inc., 1975.

Index

Accountability
  application in education, 4, 5, 48
  planning for, 6, 7
  of student, 5
  of teacher, 5, 6
Behavior(s). *See* Domains of learning
Binet, Alfred, 46
Bloom, Benjamin, et al., 29, 32, 39, 98, 99,
  123, 155
Communication skills, 117, 150, 151
Competencies
  in affective domain, 73–76
  analysis by domains of learning, 29,
    72–78
  analysis by dominant and secondary
    domains, 30, 31
  in cognitive domain, 72, 73
  definition of, 17, 18, 22
  in psychomotor domain, 76–78
  samples of, 22, 24, 25
  subcompetencies, 18, 59, 79
Criteria
  for evaluation, 78, 79
  for human relations, 21, 22
  for nursing tasks, 19
Curriculum
  committee and duties, 91–95
  definition of, 89, 90
  as implementation of philosophy, 2, 3
  learning activities in, 96, 97, 104, 105
  objectives of, 90, 91
  planning, 6
  sequence in, 98
Domains of learning
  affective, 29
    levels within, 37
    in nursing, 38, 39
  cognitive, 29
    levels within, 30
    in nursing, 33
    observable and nonobservable, 32–39
  psychomotor, 29
    levels within, 34
    in nursing, 34–36
Evaluation. *See also* Tests
  comparison of criterion-referenced and
    norm-referenced, 45–50, 186
  criteria for, 78, 79
  criterion-referenced
    formative, 187
    summative, 187
  definition of, 43
  devices, selection of, 45, 50, 51
  domain-referenced grading, 186–89
  feedback from, 4, 44, 49, 95, 119, 123,
    126

  measurement, comparison with, 43
  norm-referenced, uses of, 186
  observation, 65, 66
  purposes of, 44, 45, 185
  reliability of, 45, 46
  validity of, 45
Grading, 185–89. *See also* Evaluation
Gronlund, Norman E., 187, 191
Institutions
  board of trustees, 2
  educational, 1, 2
  philosophy of, 2
Jarolimek, John, and Clifford Foster, 125
Keller, Fred S., 134
Krathwohl, David R., et al., 37, 98
Lapp, Diane, et al., 114
Learner(s)
  individual needs of, 131
  receptivity, overcoming barriers to,
    118–20
  role of, 144
Learning
  activities, selection of, 96, 136–56
    sequence of, 97, 98, 103
  aids and resources for, 167–79
  categories or domains, 29
  definition of, 1
  factors that influence, 121–26
  instruction, individualized, 132–35
  motivation for, 122
  objectives, 8
  outcomes, 3–5
  process of, 111–12
    concept formation, 112–13
    perception, 112
    transfer, 114
Mager, Robert F., 71, 98
Nursing care study, 63–65
Objectives
  behavioral, 50
    definition of, 4, 71
    elements of, 98
    evaluation, in relation to, 50
    pretest and posttest to measure, 81, 185
    steps in writing, 171–78
  criterion- and goal-referenced
    advantages of, 8
    definition of, 5
Partnership
  in criterion- or goal-referenced
  instruction, 8
  in teacher-learner relationship, 7, 8, 116,
    118
Patient's bill of rights, 19–21
Skills. *See* Domains of learning
Taba, Hilda

method of identifying tasks, 14
method of sequencing questions, 13, 99
research, 99
nursing, identification of, 13–16
standards for, 19, 21
Teachers of nursing
activities of, 115
preparation of, 115, 116
qualities of, 116–18
role of, 114, 116
Teaching
aids and resources for, 167–79
audiovisual, 173–78
visual, 168–72
definition of, 1
instruction
criterion- or goal-referenced, 8
individualized, 132–35

lesson plans for, 156–59
microlesson, 160–62
sample, 159
methods of, 137–56
process, 1, 3
strategies to meet individual needs, 131
Dalton plan, 131
Winnetka plan, 131
Tests
criterion-referenced, 47–50, 187
reliability of, 45, 46
criterion-referenced and norm-referenced,
compared, 45–50, 186
grading, basis for, 54, 185
pretest and posttest, 81
types of, 51–66
validity of, 45, 46
Weigand, James E., ed., 57